MCQs and Short Notes in Psychiatry

MCQs and Short Notes in Psychiatry

Alistair S. Burns MB ChB MRCP MRCPsych DHMSA
Research Worker and Honorary Senior Registrar

Anthony S. David MB ChB MRCP MRCPsych
Research Worker and Honorary Senior Registrar

Michael Farrell MB Bch MRCP MRCPsych
Senior Registrar

Institute of Psychiatry and Maudsley Hospital, London

Foreword by **Robin M. Murray** MPhil MD FRCP FRCPsych
Dean, Institute of Psychiatry

WRIGHT
London   Boston   Singapore   Sydney   Toronto   Wellington

Wright
is an imprint of Butterworth Scientific

First published, 1988

© Butterworth & Co. (Publishers) Ltd, 1988

British Library Cataloguing in Publication Data

Burns, Alistair S.
 MCQs and short notes in psychiatry
 1. Medicine. Psychiatry – Questions & answers
 I. Title II. David, Anthony S. III. Farrell Michael
 616.89′0076

 ISBN 0-7236-0938-1

Library of Congress Cataloging in Publication Data

Burns, Alistair S.
 MCQs and short notes in psychiatry.
 1. Psychiatry—Examinations, questions, etc.
 I. David, Anthony S. II. Farrell, Michael.
 III. Title. [DNLM: 1. Psychiatry—examination
 questions. 2. Psychiatry—outlines. WM 18 B967m]
 RC457.B87   1988   616.89′0076   88-5673
 ISBN 0-7236-0938-1

Photoset by Butterworths Litho Preparation Department
Printed and bound in Great Britain by Butler and Tanner, Frome, Somerset

FOREWORD

The distillation of the concepts underlying psychiatry into the rigid MCQ format rarely does justice to the fascinating complexity of our subject. Nevertheless, mastery of the MRCPsych exam is a prerequisite of a career in psychiatry, and the Royal College, rightly or wrongly, believes that knowledge is most effectively tested by MCQs and by short notes. The existence of the MRCPsych in its present form, therefore, means that it is the duty of those of us who are involved in postgraduate teaching to ensure that our trainees obtain the MRCPsych in as painless a manner as possible. Only then can they devote themselves to more beneficial pursuits.

Perhaps because of their Celtic origins, Doctors Burns, David and Farrell have been able to peer through the swirling mists of fashionable exam techniques to produce a route map to help stragglers on their way to the psychiatric equivalent of the Holy Grail. The reader is provided with more than the enigma of a true or false answer. Instead, he or she is given a brief explanation of why the question was asked plus some broader information in order to guide further study. Contemporary issues in psychiatry, some of which have not yet permeated the standard textbooks, are dealt with concisely. Exam candidates will find this book useful in avoiding the traps laid for them by the Royal College. They may even learn a few facts relevant to the care of their patients and the advancement of their subject.

ROBIN M. MURRAY
Dean, Institute of Psychiatry

PREFACE

The prospective candidate for the Royal College of Psychiatrists exam is confronted by a bewildering array of study aids. Recent years have witnessed a small explosion in the number of publications specifically designed to help assimilate the basic facts required. The mainstay of assessment of factual knowledge is the MCQ. This has the advantage of being an accurate reflection of a candidate's knowledge and can be marked objectively. It is thus an important weapon in the examiner's armamentarium. The essay question requires skills of logical presentation and expression of ideas. Recent changes in the examination have included the addition of a clinical section to part I and also short answer questions to part II. The latter are considered intermediate between the rigid dichotomy of the MCQ and the eclectic liberalism of the essay.

This modest addition to the psychiatric literature is an attempt to mirror both changes in the exam and provide an up-to-date digest of current psychiatric thinking. MCQs and short notes on the scientific basis of psychiatry and major clinical specialties are provided with answers. Topics as diverse as neuroimaging, AIDS, history, cognitive therapy, molecular genetics, child abuse and neuroendocrinology are included. It may help the fledgling psychiatric matador to take the bull by the horns. It is not designed to be an in-depth reflection of the entire field but a basis from which the candidate may test himself, highlighting areas to be studied more thoroughly.

We are most grateful to our many teachers and especially to Dr Robin Murray for his thoughtful foreword.

A.S.B.
A.S.D.
M.F.
London

HOW TO USE THIS BOOK

The main purpose of this book is to act as a basis for further revision and to highlight deficits in the candidates' knowledge. The MCQs are placed in sections in order to focus on a particular subject which should stimulate further reading. As with all MCQ practice, it is best to run through the questions, noting down the answers and checking them afterwards. The standard notation is used: T = true and F = false. In the exam, a wrong answer is penalized with a minus mark, a correct answer gains one mark and an unanswered question gains nothing. The candidate alone can judge whether he or she should guess or not and this can be discovered only with practice.

The short notes (officially known as Short Answer Questions) test knowledge on a particular subject in more detail. They are a new addition to the exam and are considered as complementary to the MCQ. There is a selection of twenty covering a range of topics which could conceivably be included in the exam.

The trick of passing the exam is not so much encyclopaedic knowledge but an awareness of what topics may be asked. This book should be used as a guide to the range of subjects and questions which await the candidate.

CONTENTS

Basic Sciences

Clinical Psychiatry

NEUROANATOMY

1. **The corpus callosum**
    A:　is part of the limbic system
    B:　may be congenitally absent
    C:　consists largely of unmyelinated fibres
    D:　if transected, gives rise to astereognosis
    E:　forms part of the Papez circuit

2. **The interstitial cells of the CNS**
    A:　are of mesodermal origin
    B:　include astrocytes
    C:　occur in similar numbers to neurones
    D:　are known as mesoglia
    D:　form part of the blood-brain barrier

3. **The following are parts of the extrapyramidal system:**
    A:　caudate nucleus
    B:　dentate nucleus
    C:　red nucleus
    D:　Reiter's nucleus
    E:　internal capsule

1.

A: **F** The limbic system is a *functional* rather than anatomical unit. It consists of: primary olfactory cortex, septal cortex (just below the genu of the corpus callosum), hippocampus, cingulate gyrus, subcortical limbic nuclei which includes the septal nuclei and the amygdala. A favourite part 1 question.

B: **T** Agenesis can occur and this may be a fortuitous CT scan finding.

C: **F**

D: **T** But only in certain circumstances i.e. naming of objects placed in the left hand, with the subject blind-folded!

E: **F** Another functional unit which links the limbic system and the neocortex. Considered now as out-dated but still features in examination questions.

2.

A: **F** They are of ectodermal origin. Mesoglia (connective tissue cells) are of mesodermal origin.

B: **T** Astrocytes and oligodendrocytes are the two main types of interstitial cells.

C: **F** They are ten times more common than neurones.

D: **F** They are known as neuroglia.

E: **T** They almost completely surround the capillaries and thus, in conjunction with vascular endothelium form the 'gliovascular membrane'.

3.

A: **T** The basal ganglia are part of the extrapyramidal system and consist of the lentiform nucleus (putamen and globus pallidus) and caudate nucleus. The other main part of the extrapyramidal system is the cerebellum.

B: **T** Part of the cerebellum with major connections to the thalamus.

C: **T** The brain stem nuclei are an important part of the system and include the substantia nigra, midbrain and tectal nuclei, and the lateral vestibular nucleus (Reiter's nucleus).

D: **T**

E: **F** This is the area through which the pyramidal fibres pass from the cortex to spinal cord.

4. **The following structures develop from the prosencephalon:**
A: rhinencephalon
B: basal ganglia
C: metencephalon
D: cerebellum
E: thalamus

5. **Parts of the Papez circuit include:**
A: hypothalamus
B: cingulate gyrus
C: thalamus
D: fornix
E: amygdala

6. **In the blood supply to the brain**
A: the posterior communicating artery connects anterior and posterior cerebral arteries
B: the anterior communicating artery connects both anterior cerebral arteries
C: pontine arteries come from the vertebral arteries
D: the right basilar artery supplies the right lobe of the cerebellum
E: the posterior inferior cerebellar artery is a branch of the vertebral artery

7. **The right cerebral hemisphere is specialised in**
A: facial recognition
B: musical appreciation
C: prosody
D: processing emotions
E: analytic thought

4.
A: T The primitive forebrain (prosencephalon) gives rise to those parts of the cerebral hemispheres known as the rhinencephalon which include the olfactory bulbs and lobes, the basal ganglia and pallidum. In addition, a part of the prosencephalon remains in the mid-line and gives rise to the thalamus, hypothalamus and epithalamus. The metencephalon arises from the hindbrain and cerebellum, medulla and pons are part of it.
B: T
C: F
D: F
E: T

5.
A: F The Papez circuit was first described in 1937 as the possible basis for emotional behaviour. It links the limbic system with the neocortex through the cingulate gyrus. The circuit consists of the hippocampus, mamillary body, thalamus, cingulate gyrus and then back to the hippocampus.
B: T
C: T
D: F
E: F

6.
A: F It connects middle and posterior cerebral arteries.
B: T
C: F They come from the basilar artery
D: F There is only one basilar artery, formed by the two vertebrals.
E: T

7.
A: T Right parietal. Prosopagnosia (failure of facial recognition) is usually due to bilateral lesions.
B: T Melody is affected more than appreciation of tempo following right hemisphere lesions.
C: T The 'musical quality' of speech.
D: T Particularly facial expression, but this is debated.
E: F This is said to be the preferred mode of processing for the left hemisphere. The right uses a more gestalt/holistic mode.

8. **The hypothalamus plays a part in the control of**
   A: satiety
   B: gender identity
   C: fluid balance
   D: anti diuretic hormone (ADH) secretion
   E: memory

9. **The pineal gland**
   A: receives fibres from the retina
   B: is the site of the 'biological clock'
   C: is innervated by fibres from the superior cervical ganglion
   D: secretes melanin
   E: is the seat of the soul

10. **The following pass through the foramen magnum:**
   A: anterior spinal artery
   B: vertebral artery
   C: basilar artery
   D: spinal accessory nerve
   E: vagus nerve

11. **The trigeminal nerve**
   A: supplies sensation to the cornea through its second division
   B: innervates the muscles of mastication
   C: supplies sensation to the face and angle of the jaw
   D: may be damaged by a tumour in the jugular foramen
   E: carries pain and temperature fibres which form the quinto-thalamic tract

8.
A: **T** Ventromedial nucleus. Ablation of the lateral nucleus produces anorexia.
B: **F** Sexual behaviour is controlled by the anterior hypothalamus.
C: **T**
D: **T** ADH is secreted by the supraoptic nuclei and then transported to and released by the posterior pituitary gland.
E: **F** Limbic structures.

9.
A: **T** Via fibres passing through the suprachiasmatic nucleus (SCN).
B: **F** Although the pineal gland plays a role, it is the SCN which is the location of the so-called biological clock. Ablation of the SCN leads to abolition of most circadian rhythms.
C: **T** Sympathetic innervation.
D: **F** Melatonin.
E: **T** According to the philosopher Descartes!

10.
A: **T** This arises from the vertebral arteries in the foramen magnum. The two vessels join to become a single artery opposite the odontoid peg.
B: **T**
C: **F** The two vertebral arteries pass through the foramen before joining to form the basilar artery.
D: **T** This is the 11th cranial nerve and innervates the sternomastoid muscle and upper part of trapezius.
E: **F** Exits through the jugular foramen.

11.
A: **F** Supplies sensation to the cornea by its first division, the ophthalmic. Loss of upper facial sensation with intact corneal sensation is likely to be functional.
B: **T**
C: **F** Not the angle of the jaw which is supplied by the C2 and C3 via the greater auricular nerve.
D: **F** Would be damaged by a tumour in the cerebello-pontine angle.
E: **T**

NEUROCHEMISTRY

12. **Gamma amino butyric acid (GABA)**
    A: is the principal inhibitory neurotransmitter
    B: is formed from the decarboxylation of α-ketoglutarate
    C: if deficient in the CNS, may lead to convulsions
    D: is facilitated by benzodiazepines
    E: is present in the brain in greater concentrations than noradrenaline

13. **Glycine:**
    A: has an effect on presynaptic membranes
    B: brain concentrations are about 25% of spinal cord concentrations
    C: hypopolarises motor neurones
    D: is a potent inhibitory neurotransmitter
    E: strychnine competes for the same receptor

14. **Substance P**
    A: is particularly concentrated in the intestine and nervous tissue
    B: exists in high concentrations in the hypothalamus
    C: is not found in the spinal cord
    D: may be involved in neurotransmission
    E: is most likely to be an inhibitory neurotransmitter

15. **The following areas are recognised to contain noradrenaline:**
    A: hippocampus
    B: locus coeruleus
    C: cingulate gyrus
    D: thalamus
    E: substantia nigra

12.
A: T
B: F Transamination of α-ketoglutarate.
C: T May be precipitated by vitamin B6 deficiency, because glutamate decarboxylase, involved in GABA synthesis, is pyridoxine dependent.
D: T Benzodiazepines attach to specific sites which enhance GABA receptor binding. GABA is also potentiated by ethanol and barbiturates.
E: T Considerably so.

13.
A: F An amino acid which has a powerful inhibitory neurotransmitter effect in the spinal cord - effects post-synaptic membranes.
B: T
C: F It hyperpolarises them.
D: T
E: T

14.
A: T First observed in 1934, now known to be a peptide.
B: T Also in putamen, caudate and globus pallidus.
C: F In lower concentrations than brain but is present.
D: T Found in fibres signalling pain (slow conducting, non-myelinated fibres).
E: F Most likely to be excitatory.

15.
A: T
B: T This is the main adrenergic nucleus.
C: F Cingulate cortex contains noradrenaline whereas the cingulate *gyrus* contains dopamine.
D: T
E: F Dopamine (the immediate precursor of noradrenaline).

16. With regard to phenylalanine metabolism:
A: phenylalanine hydroxylase oxidises phenylalanine to tyrosine
B: phenylalanine hydroxylase deficiency occurs in 1 in 10,000 births
C: in phenylketonuria, serum phenylalanine increases ten fold
D: tyrosine uptake is increased with excess phenylalanine
E: phenylpyruvic acid is produced in phenylketonuria

17. Hypocalcaemia is associated with
A: intracranial calcification
B: artificial infant feeds
C: fits
D: psychosis
E: mental retardation

18. With regard to cystine metabolism:
A: cystathionine synthetase activity is almost non-existent in homocystinuria
B: cystathione is a direct precursor of methionine
C: cystathione is greatly increased in concentration in homocystinuria
D: mental retardation always occurs in homocystinuria
E: two molecules of homocysteine join to form homocystine

16.

A: T Tyrosine is then metabolised to DOPA, dopamine and adrenaline or into melanin.

B: T Classical phenylketonuria.

C: F It is increased 30 fold, urine phenylalanine is increased 10-30 times.

D: F Tyrosine uptake is decreased hence light pigmentation occurs because tyrosine is not available for metabolism into melanin.

E: T Along with other abnormal metabolites such as phenylacetic acid and phenyllactic acid.

17.

A: T Seen on CT scan. Other causes include, infection (esp toxoplasmosis), arterio-venous malformations and tumour (esp oligodendroglioma).

B: T Particularly those high in phosphate.

C: T Also causes muscle twitches and tetany.

D: T

E: T May be part of the pseudohypoparathyroid syndrome.

18.

A: T This is the enzyme which manufactures cystathione from its precursor homocystine. Homocystine therefore builds up excessively in the enzymes absence. The normal pathway is homocystine cystathionine cystine. Homocystinuria is the inborn error of metabolism affecting the production of this sulphur containing amino acid and is a relatively common autosomal recessive condition, second only in frequency to phenylketonuria.

B: F Methionine is metabolised to homocystine and thence cystathione.

C: F Absent. It is a normal constituent of brain.

D: F Often occurs but not always (questions with 'always' in them are 'always' wrong). Skeletal and cardiac abnormalities, epilepsy and liver degeneration may occur.

E: T

19. Dimethyltryptamine (DMT)
A: is a naturally occuring psychotomimetic
B: is found in normal subjects' urine
C: is found in increased amounts in urine during acute psychotic episodes
D: correlates with daily fluctuations in mood
E: causes inward withdrawal as well as hallucinations

20. The amine hypothesis of affective disorder is supported by
A: the observation that reserpine improved depression
B: the amine uptake inhibition caused by tricyclic antidepressants
C: the antidepressant action of cocaine
D: low urinary levels of 3-methoxy 4-hydroxyphenylglycol (MHPG) in depressives
E: alterations in homovanillic acid (HVA) levels in depressives

19.

A: T It is produced by the transmethylation of tryptamine a psychotomimetic four times as potent as mescaline.

B: T

C: T This occurs transiently but is a non-specific finding in psychotic illnesses in general. It is also found in patients with liver disease.

D: F

E: T This led to its promise as a good model for schizophrenia.

20.

A: F Reserpine was one of the early anti-hypertensive drugs which caused depression in up to 15% patients - it was never reported to cause mania.

B: T Theoretically, this increases the amount of amines in the synaptic cleft.

C: F Cocaine is a psychoactive amine but does not have a clinical antidepressant effect.

D: T MHPG is a major metabolite of noradrenaline.

E: F There is great variability in the levels of HVA, the main metabolite of dopamine, in depression.

NEUROPHYSIOLOGY

21. The following occurs in the neuronal action potential:
A: the cell membrane slowly becomes permeable
B: there is a great influx of sodium into the cell
C: the action potential lasts about 10 milliseconds
D: the inside of the cell changes from positive to negative
E: potassium enters the cell

22. The following are true about neuro-muscular transmission:
A: may produce inhibition of the muscle cell
B: one neuronal action potential can give rise to several muscle action potentials
C: d-tubocurarine blocks the action potential
D: acetylcholine levels may fall in the junctional area with repeated stimulation
E: acetylcholine is only effective in the junctional area

23. The following are true of the EEG:
A: alpha rhythm arises predominantly from the frontal cortex
B: beta rhythm has a frequency of 8-12Hz
C: a flat trace is diagnostic of brain death
D: with age, fast activity becomes more prominent
E: rapid eye movement (REM) sleep is devoid of spindle activity

21.
A: F At the onset of the action potential, the cell membranes suddenly becomes permeable to ions.
B: T The increased permeability leads to sodium influx.
C: F Lasts 1-2 msecs.
D: F From -70 to $+40$ mVolts
E: F

22.
A: F *Never* inhibitory in mammals.
B: F Always one-to-one, a simple synapse.
C: F Blocks the action of Ach. on the muscle but does not effect the action potential.
D: T With increased activity. Levels do increase around the muscle fibre.
E: T

23.
A: F Alpha is a parieto-occipital rhythm.
B: F Beta is 12-14Hz, alpha is 8-11Hz, theta is 4-7Hz and delta is 1-4Hz.
C: F The EEG. has no place in the criteria for brain death, but may be used to support a clinical diagnosis.
D: T
E: T REM or paradoxical sleep is accompanied by hypotonia with loss of stretch reflexes, variation in heart and respiratory rate, penile erection (except in organic impotence) and a low-voltage EEG, without spindle activity (14Hz bursts occuring in deep, non-REM sleep).

24. The following have been demonstrated in dementia:
A: slowing of peripheral motor nerve conduction
B: slowing of peripheral sensory nerve conduction
C: improved peripheral nerve conduction with vitamin B complex supplements
D: delayed cortical somatosensory evoked potentials
E: the degree of slowing of peripheral nerve conduction correlates with the severity of dementia

25. Event-related potentials
A: are obtained by taking a series of EEG recordings and averaging them together
B: are termed 'early' if they occur within the first 10 msec
C: occuring after 300msec are uninfluenced by attention
D: early potentials are not present if the subject is anaesthetised
E: may utilise the 'oddball paradigm'

26. The galvanic skin response (GSR)
A: forms the basis of the lie detector test
B: is a sensitive measure of anxiety
C: shows decreased arousal in chronic schizophrenia
D: is controlled by the limbic system ipsilaterally
E: is slow to habituate in some schizophrenics

24.
A: T This affects motor conduction only and is not present in age-matched cognitively normal controls.
B: F
C: F No improvement after 3 months treatment in one study.
D: T As are auditory evoked potentials.
E: T The more severe the dementia, the slower the conduction and as dementia worsens, so conduction slows.

25.
A: T This 'averaging' serves to filter out 'noise' and retain the 'signal'. The potentials themselves may be in any sensory modality.
B: F It is generally agreed that patterns occurring in the first 40msec are termed 'early'. Peaks described by the convention of using 'N' or 'P' for negative and positive respectively, followed by the number denoting the time in milliseconds after the stimulus (eg P300).
C: F
D: F The early peaks are called exogenous components and are not modulated by subject factors significantly (including general anaesthesia). The P300 components are highly susceptible to internal conditions (attention, cognitive set etc) and are called the endogenous components.
E: T This is what happens when an array of similar stimuli contains an unexpected one. The P300 is enhanced using this approach.

26.
A: T An unreliable test but one used to provide evidence in a court of law in the U.S.A.
B: F It is a measure of arousal which is linked to anxiety but less specific. It also includes fear, anger and other mental states.
C: F It is increased. It is believed that some negative symptoms of schizophrenia are secondary strategies to reduce this hyper-arousal.
D: T Orienting response, measured in this way may be asymmetrical in some schizophrenics, pointing to (left) limbic dysfunction.
E: T Related to increased baseline arousal.

27. In the human adult brain
A: oxygen consumption is highest in the basal ganglia
B: low blood glucose slows brain metabolism
C: glucose is the principal source of energy
D: the respiratory quotient is 1.0
E: glucose utilisation decreases with age

28. The following increase cerebral blood flow:
A: carotid sinus massage
B: stellate ganglion blockade
C: polycythaemia
D: increased CO_2 concentration
E: decreased intracranial pressure

29. In the measurement of cerebral blood flow (CBF)
A: Kety and Schmidt developed a technique using xenon-133
B: xenon-133 can be injected or inhaled to assess CBF
C: Kety found CBF to be decreased in schizophrenic patients compared to controls
D: using xenon-133 in normals, there is relatively more blood flow to the posterior lobes
E: tracers require to cross the blood-brain barrier

27.
A: F Highest in the cortex and cerebellum.
B: T High blood glucose has no direct effect (until diabetic coma supervenes).
C: T This is the same as foetal brain but the adult brain synthesises less protein and lipid.
D: T This suggests that the tissues use carbohydrate exclusively.
E: T PET scan studies suggest that this is the case.

28.
A: T Increases vagal tone.
B: T Causes a decrease in sympathetic stimulation. Beta-blockers (eg propranolol) do the opposite and may therefore be used to treat migraine.
C: F This decreases cerebral blood flow, often by over 50%.
D: T A 5-7% increase in CO_2 concentration may induce a 75% increase in cerebral blood flow. Mechanical hyperventilation may be used by the neurosurgeon to reduce intracranial pressure.
E: T Intracranial CSF pressure leads to resistance to blood flow.

29.
A: F This was by Ingvar in the 1960's. Kety and Schmidt developed the nitrous oxide technique in the 1940's.
B: T The original experiments involved intracarotid injection - then inhalation was used.
C: F No difference was found in these early experiments.
D: F To the frontal lobes - the reverse pattern was found in schizophrenia.
E: T Thus, they equilibrate with brain parenchyma and so distribution can easily be assessed.

NEUROPHARMACOLOGY

30. The endogenous opioids
A: bind to the same receptor as morphine
B: consist of metencephalin and β endorphin
C: can cause muscular rigidity when in excess
D: can be excitatory
E: are increased in depressed patients with chronic pain

31. Carbamazepine may be useful in the treatment of
A: petit mal epilepsy
B: rapid cycling bipolar affective disorder
C: trigeminal neuralgia
D: aggressive behaviour in the mentally handicapped
E: benign familial essential tremor

32. Benzodiazepines
A: act via GABAergic pathways
B: have at least 2 types of receptors in the brain
C: cannot be displaced from their binding sites by nicotinamide
D: reduce fast α activity
E: can increase goal-directed behaviour

30.

A: T The morphine receptor was identified through the specificity of the antagonist, naloxone. Endogenous substances were found to bind to the same receptors.

B: F Met-encephalin is the same as part of the bigger substance β endorphin. Met and leu-encephalins are the two opioids.

C: F The so called 'natural neuroleptics'.

D: T In the hippocampus, where no receptors have been identified.

E: F Some evidence that they may be increased in deliberate self-cutters.

31.

A: F Favoured for focal epilepsy but can be used in grand mal epilepsy.

B: T Recently discovered therapeutic possibility, either with or without lithium but requires more research.

C: T Even in the absence of epilepsy. Slows nerve conduction.

D: T

E: F Treated with propranolol. Also responds favourably to alcohol!

32.

A: T As do barbiturates and alcohol

B: T Substances related to β carboline may be endogenous ligands which bind to these receptors.

C: F

D: F Increases it. Nevertheless, they increase the seizure threshold.

E: T Like alcohol, their anxiety reducing action may lead to increased aggression and other examples of disinhibition.

33. Tardive dyskinesia may be caused by
A: chlordiazepoxide
B: haloperidol
C: benzhexol
D: lithium
E: sulpiride

34. Ectopic ACTH secretion may result in
A: a positive dexamethasone suppression test
B: Cushing's syndrome
C: depression
D: mania
E: fatigue

35. In the metabolism of alcohol
A: ethanol is metabolised to acetic acid and then acetaldehyde
B: disulfiram (Antabuse) inhibits acetaldehyde dehydrogenase
C: calcium carbimide citrate decreases the effect of disulfiram
D: the principle pathway is via alcohol dehydrogenase
E: in chronic alcoholism, microsomal ethanol oxidation decreases

33.

A: F

B: T   Virtually all neuroleptic agents have been implicated in causing tardive dyskinesia (TD). This includes drugs not specifically used in psychiatry such as metoclopramide.

C: T   This is an anticholinergic drug. These may precipitate and worsen TD though they alleviate acute dystonias and some cases of tardive dystonia.

D: T   Lithium has some central dopamine blocking activity.

E: F   This is a new specific D2 receptor blocker which has not been associated with TD, yet!

34.

A: T   Exceptions do occur. Dexamethasone is a synthetic steroid which, in normal people inhibits endogenous ACTH secretion and therefore cortisol by negative feedback. Carroll *et al*, ((1981) *Arch Gen Psych;* 38:15-22) showed that a modification of the test namely giving 1mg at 11.30 pm and then measuring plasma cortisol at 4 pm and 11 pm the following day, revealed nonsuppression (cortisol levels > 5μgm/dl) in the majority of severely depressed patients.

B: T

C: T

D: T   A variety of psychiatric manifestations have been noted and include affective and schizophreniform psychoses.

E: T   Due to hypokalaemia.

35.

A: F   Acetaldehyde is produced from ethanol and is then itself broken down to acetic acid.

B: T   Thus increasing the hang-over effects which are produced by acetaldehyde.

C: F

D: T   An NAD dependent enzyme.

E: F   It increases due to endoplasmic activation.

36. The dopamine hypothesis of schizophrenia is supported by the observation that
A: amphetamines may cause a paranoid psychosis
B: mescaline causes hallucinations
C: Parkinson's disease and schizophrenia are associated
D: the rise in prolactin level following neuroleptic drugs is the same in normals as in schizophrenics
E: the antipsychotic action of neuroleptics is closely related to their capacity to block dopamine receptors

37. The neuroleptic malignant syndrome
A: is a form of lymphoma induced by long term neuroleptic treatment
B: is an extrapyramidal syndrome
C: is an idiosyncratic response to neuroleptics
D: may be treated with bromocriptine
E: may be treated with dantrolene

38. The following antidepressants characteristically cause sedation:
A: amitriptyline
B: nortriptyline
C: mianserin
D: doxepin
E: desipramine.

36.

A: **T** Amphetamine psychosis, occurring after prolonged and heavy abuse may be indistinguishable from paranoid schizophrenia. Amphetamine is a catecholamine/dopamine agonist.

B: **F** Mescaline has a similar structure to noradrenaline; the psychedelic phenomena produced by it are different from schizophrenia in terms of affect and also the predominantly visual hallucinations.

C: **F** There is no association. Parkinson's disease (a nigro-striatal dopamine deficiency) was once thought to be incompatible with schizophrenia (a putative mesolimbic functional dopamine excess). This has been shown not to be the case and implies that the two dopaminergic systems are to some extent independent.

D: **F** Dopamine inhibits the release of prolactin (tuberoinfundibular pathway). The similarity in the rise of prolactin following neuroleptics (dopamine antagonists) goes against the dopamine hypothesis.

E: **T** This is the most convincing evidence to date.

37.

A: **F**

B: **T** Extreme rigidity and immobility, thought to be due to total dopamine blockade.

C: **T**

D: **T** A dopamine agonist

E: **T** A muscle relaxant used to treat the hyperpyrexia and rhabdomyolysis which may be fatal.

38.

A: **T** Correlates with anti-histamine receptor affinity. Sedative antidepressants may be useful where anxiety and insomnia are prominent.

B: **F** Believed to have a 'therapeutic window', that is levels above (and below) the therapeutic level may not be effective.

C: **T**

D: **T**

E: **F** Note also that some MAOIs such as tranylcypromine may be stimulant reflecting a similar structure to amphetamines.

39. With lithium therapy
A: absorption of a dose is complete in 8 hours
B: peak plasma levels occur 6 hours after absorption
C: a third is excreted within 12 hours
D: decreased salt intake decreases the excretion of lithium
E: levels are increased by administration of carbonic anhydrase

40. The following may be prescribed for a 50 year-old man with impaired liver function:
A: imipramine
B: phenelzine
C: primidone
D: diazepam
E: phenytoin

39.
A: **T** This takes 6-8 hours.
B: **F** Occurs ½-2 hours after ingestion
C: **T**
D: **F** If increased sodium intake occurs, this will result in increased excretion of sodium. The reduced renal tubular reabsorption of sodium will increase lithium excretion.
E: **F** Levels are unaffected by carbonic anhydrase. Other diuretics may increase lithium levels and may cause toxicity in the elderly.

40.
A: **T** Tricyclics are preferable to MAOIs but sedative effects are increased.
B: **F** This may cause idiosyncratic hepatotoxicity.
C: **F** May precipitate coma and should be avoided if possible.
D: **F** In general benzodiazepines should be avoided as all can precipitate coma but if one must be used, the shorter acting oxazepam is preferable. If chlormethiazole (Heminevrin) must be used, its dose should be lowered considerably.
E: **T** Can be used if dose is reduced and levels are monitored regularly.

PSYCHOLOGY

41. The following tests are used by clinical psychologists to test memory:
- A: paired associates test
- B: Wisconsin Card Sort test
- C: Gollin's figures
- D: proverb interpretation
- E: Rey-Osterrieth figure

42. The concept of learned helplessness
- A: was described by Seligman
- B: is based on experiments with rats
- C: results when an attitude of helplessness is reinforced by social rewards
- D: does not affect victims of torture
- E: is incompatible with Brown and Harris' social theories of depression

43. Introversion
- A: was a term introduced by Jung
- B: was used by Eysenck as a dimension of personality
- C: is associated with obsessionality
- D: if high, makes an individual slower to condition
- E: correlates with low cortical arousal

41.

A: T

B: F   A frontal lobe test of the ability to change sorting strategies

C: F   A parietal function test

D: F   Sometimes used as a 'bedside' test of thought disorder but probably more related to education than psychopathology.

E: T   A complex geometrical figure which must be copied directly first, then from memory. It is therefore a test of visual memory.

42.

A: T   In 1975

B: F   Dogs! The experiment involved giving electric shocks to dogs, who learned to avoid them by jumping over a barrier. When this escape was denied the animal, it lapsed into an apathetic, helpless state which remained even after the means of escape was reinstated.

C: F   This is more akin to the sick role.

D: F   Frequently affects them.

E: F   It may be argued that persistent social deprivation, of the sort described by Brown and Harris in their studies of the 'Social Origins of Depression', (1978, Tavistock Publications, London) causes a kind of learned helplessness.

43.

A: T

B: T   The dimensions are introversion-extraversion and stable-neurotic.

C: T   Obsessionals are said to be neurotic introverts. Psychopaths are said to be neurotic extraverts.

D: T

E: F   The opposite is true.

44. In classical conditioning

   A: extinction is the fading of the response to an unconditioned stimulus with time
   B: backward conditioning is where the conditioned stimulus precedes the unconditioned stimulus
   C: chaining is the process whereby a behaviour is broken down into its components, each of which is separately reinforced
   D: stimulus generalisation does not occur
   E: may be useful in the treatment of alcoholism

45. Cognitive dissonance

   A: was described by Festinger
   B: is used by Beck's cognitive therapy to bring about change
   C: is the name of the feeling induced by double binds
   D: refers to a theory of how attitudes change
   E: is seen in schizophrenia where emotions are split from thinking

44.

A: F Extinction occurs when the conditioned stimulus (the bell in Pavlov's experiment) is given in the absence of the unconditioned stimulus (the food).

B: F

C: F Chaining describes the sequence in which the first act in a series is reinforced until it is performed reliably. Then, the contingencies are altered so that the first two acts have to be performed before reinforcement is given. This process continues until a long sequence is learned.

D: F It occurs when a conditioned response is elicited following a different but allied stimulus without specific learning. The closer the new stimulus is to the original, the greater the response.

E: T The nausea (an unconditional consequence of alcohol in a patient treated with disulfiram (Antabuse)) may follow the conditional stimulus of, for example the smell of alcohol. However, it is also the case that the nausea acts as a negative reinforcer to the undesired symptom and hence follows the operant conditioning paradigm.

45.

A: T In 1957. It refers to the feeling engendered by voluntary behaviour which is inconsistent with a persons attitudes.

B: F Aaron Beck's therapy explores maladaptive cognitions e.g. automatic negative thoughts, so that patients gradually learn new ways of evaluating themselves and events in a more positive light.

C: F The double bind was a term introduced by Gregory Bateson to describe contradictory communication patterns in families of schizophrenics.

D: T

E: F

46. Acting out
A: was originally used to describe a form of resistance during psychoanalysis.
B: is generally used to refer to impulsive anti-social or dangerous actions.
C: never has unconscious determinants.
D: can be used to describe habitual modes of behaviour related to personality rather than a specific treatment situation.
E: is closely related to countertransference.

47. The following psychological treatments are associated with names beside them:
A: Token Economy - Keynes
B: Structural family therapy - Minuchin
C: Reciprocal inhibition - Eysenck
D: Hypnotherapy - Erikson
E: Psychodrama - Hitchcock

48. The following psychological concepts are associated with the names beside them:
A: projective identification - Klein
B: splitting - Bleuler
C: dissociation - Breuer
D: EST - Cerletti & Bini
E: parapraxes - Palazzoli

46.
A: T The patient acting out that which cannot be said.
B: T
C: F Unconscious determinants are the rule.
D: T
E: F It is closely related to transference which is the term for feelings evoked in the patient towards the therapist, which relate to significant past relationships.

47.
A: F Keynes was an economist. Ayllon & Azrin developed the token economy system, a form of operant conditioning, to encourage the rehabilitation of chronically institutionalised patients.
B: T Salvador Minuchin works to restore intergenerational boundaries and the 'normal' roles of each parent, the parents as a subsystem and the sibling subsystem and hence the 'structure' of the family.
C: F Wolpe advanced this from of behavioural treatment, the pairing of an anxiety provoking stimulus with a relaxing one.
D: T Milton Erikson; not to be confused with Erik Erikson, the social psychologist.
E: F Moreno pioneered this.

48.
A: T
B: F Melanie Klein again. This refers to the splitting of the object (internalised representation of a significant figure) into good and bad parts. It is a term also used to describe dissociation.
C: F Janet. This is a mechanism found in hysteria.
D: F EST stands for Erhart Seminar Training. Cerletti & Bini discovered ECT.
E: F Freud described parapraxes, referring to slips of the tongue. Palazzoli is a member of the 'Milan School' of paradoxical family therapy.

49. A token economy is based on the following principles:
A: classical conditioning
B: reciprocal inhibition
C: extinction
D: modelling
E: social reinforcement is not sufficient to modify chronic patterns of behaviour.

50. The Yerkes-Dodson law
A: relates arousal to performance
B: forms a U-shaped curve
C: explains how bodily perceptions may produce anxiety
D: implies that anxiety may be helpful
E: explains why some people fail the M.R.C.Psych exam

51. Finger agnosia
A: is often complained of spontaneously
B: is usually produced by non-dominant parietal lesions
C: is part of Gerstmann's syndrome
D: refers exclusively to the patient's inability to recognise his own fingers
E: may be elicited by the In-Between Test

52. The placebo response
A: applies only to psychotherapy
B: is influenced by the size of tablet
C: is greater in the treatment of anxiety if the tablet is green
D: may include side effects
E: may be increased in a double blind controlled drug trial

49.
A: **F** Operant conditioning.
B: **F** This is also based on classical conditioning.
C: **T** The process whereby behaviour not rewarded is reduced,
D: **F** This is essentially learning by imitation. Though often incorporated into token economy units, it is not a basic underlying principle.
E: **F** Social reinforcement alone may be sufficient to improve, for example, motivation and self-care even if longstanding.

50.
A: **T**
B: **F** The law states that performance will improve as arousal increases up to a point after which a further increase in arousal reduces performance. When represented graphically this forms an inverted U-shaped curve.
C: **F** This is the James-Lange theory of anxiety
D: **T**
E: **T**

51.
A: **F** Only very rarely
B: **F** Usually dominant parietal/occipital lobe or angular gyrus lesions - occasionally non-dominant.
C: **T** The full syndrome consists of finger agnosia, dysgraphia, dyscalculia and right/left disorientation.
D: **F** Refers to an inability to recognise either their own or an examiner's fingers.
E: **T** The subject is asked the number of fingers in between two touched on their hand.

52.
A: **F** Any treatment has a placebo component.
B: **T** Very small or very large tablets are most effective.
C: **T** And yellow are best for depression!
D: **T**
E: **T** Because the tablets will be administered with equal faith and enthusiasm.

MISCELLANEOUS I

53. **The following apply to Positron Emission Tomography (PET):**
    A: Fluorine[18] is a commonly used isotope
    B: Methylspiperone binds to dopamine receptors
    C: increased activity has been shown in the frontal lobes in schizophrenia
    D: increased activity has been shown in the parietal lobes in Alzheimer's disease
    E: asymmetry in temporal lobe activity has been demonstrated during panic attacks

54. **Nuclear Magnetic Resonance (NMR)**
    A: is useful for imaging plaques in multiple sclerosis
    B: is useful for imaging plaques in Alzheimer's disease
    C: takes about 20 minutes to perform
    D: has demonstrated more abnormalities in schizophrenia than CT scans
    E: is useful in the diagnosis of Binswanger's disease

55. **In statistics, the following are correct:**
    A: The scores of one population: 1,2,3 & 4 correlate with those of another: 2,4,6 & 8 giving an r value of 1
    B: A two-tailed test is more likely to give a significant value than a one-tailed test
    C: The F test compares the variance in 2 populations
    D: The Student's t test is appropriate only if the F ratio is not significant
    E: Cronbach's α coefficient is used to measure the internal consistency of a scale

53.
A: T
B: T PET images are produced by labelling isotopes which are attached to: blood proteins, thereby showing blood flow; glucose, giving an indication of metabolic activity; receptor sites, to show quantitative differences between experimental groups or asymmetries in individuals.
C: F 'Hypofrontality' has been a repeated finding, especially in chronic patients.
D: F Decreased activity has been reported in the parietal lobes. This is in line with CT scan data in which decreased density in the parietal region has been shown to predict a rapid downhill course.
E: T Increased right sided activity has been found in one study. Patients with panic attacks who did not have an attack during the procedure showed no abnormality.

54.
A: T Particularly useful. Sclerotic plaques are not seen on CT scans.
B: F Microscopic silver staining plaques of amyloid, present in increased amounts in Alzheimer's disease. Also increased to a lesser extent in normal ageing.
C: F Nearer 90 minutes.
D: F
E: T This is a sub-acute subcortical hypertensive encephalopathy with characteristic periventricular oedema, another abnormality for which NMR is best at detecting.

55.
A: T This is why various weighting procedures are sometimes used such as the weighted kappa for test-retest reliability estimates.
B: F A two-tailed test is applied when for example the effect of a drug on performance is studied and the investigators do not specify whether it may be improved or impaired. The threshold of significance must therefore be raised.
C: T
D: T If the variance (spread around the mean) of 2 populations differs widely (i.e. the F ratio is significant) then a non-parametric test such as the Mann Whitney U test should be used.
E: T This is essentially a correlation between items on a scale.

56. **A token economy**
- A: can only be used in the hospital setting
- B: may use food as a primary reinforcer
- C: cannot be used for individuals with an IQ<50
- D: utilises Premack's principle
- E: may worsen psychotic symptoms

57. **In the history of psychiatry**
- A: Wagner von Jauregg won the Nobel prize for psychiatry
- B: Pinel introduced moral treatment
- C: Conolly was the first to suggest the humane application of physical restraint
- D: Adolf Meyer coined the term Psychobiology
- E: Freud coined the term agnosia

58. **In the recent history of psychiatry**
- A: the sedative effect of lithium was first demonstrated in mice
- B: Meduna initiated electrically induced convulsions in man
- C: the phenothiazines were first developed as antihelminthics
- D: psychosurgery was developed by Moniz
- E: Sir Aubrey Lewis was the first President of the Royal College of Psychiatrists.

56.
A: **F** Has been used by for example alcoholics anonymous to encourage non-drinking behaviour.
B: **T** Other examples include watching TV, seeing a preferred person etc.
C: **F**
D: **T** This is where behaviours of high frequency may be used as reinforcers for those of low frequency.
E: **T** Symptoms are not as amenable to this kind of treatment and may get worse initially but later returning to their previous level.

57.
A: **T** For malarial treatment of neurosyphilis!
B: **T** (1745-1826) He is associated with breaking the chains of inmates of the Saltpetriere, although he was not the first to do this.
C: **F** (1794-1866) A Victorian reformer who advocated treatment without mechanical restraints.
D: **T** (1866-1950) And introduced a unique nosology of mental disorders.
E: **T** (1856-1939) As well as publishing papers on aphasia and cerebral palsy.

58.
A: **F** Guinea pigs! All psychoactive drugs have been discovered by serendipity.
B: **F** He introduced Metrazol-supplemented chemically induced fits. This was based on the erroneous biological antagonism theory that epilepsy and psychosis were incompatible. Cerletti and Bini invented electro-shock treatment.
C: **T** And found to have sedative effects.
D: **T** Neurosurgeon, Egas Moniz (1874-1955) also a Nobel prize winner.
E: **F** Sir Martin Roth. President from 1972-5. The current President is Dr J.L.T. Birley.

59. In statistics
A: regression analysis is a form of the general linear model
B: the t test is not applicable unless the sample is strictly normally distributed
C: the null hypothesis can be accepted if $p > 0.05$
D: a distribution with a long tail to the right is positively skewed
E: the Pearson product moment correlation coefficient is a parametric test

60. In psychiatric epidemiology
A: incidence refers to the number of new cases over time
B: prevalence and point prevalence are the same
C: Kendall's tau may be used to measure the reliability of a scale
D: a target population is one which is representative of a population
E: CATEGO is a computer program used to compute the index of definition

61. In experimental design
A: a stratified sample is composed of a number of sub-samples
B: a Latin square design is used to evaluate one variable
C: probability sampling methods involve the subject being chosen on the spot by the researcher
D: quota sampling involves the subjects being selected randomly prior to the investigation
E: the independent variable is under experimental control

59.

A: T The general linear model assumes a subject's score on one variable can be derived by a combination of other variables.

B: F The test is robust to non-normality and can be used on samples not strictly normally distributed if numbers are high enough. If in doubt the Mann Whitney U test should be used.

C: F The null hypothesis can never be accepted - though if $p<0.05$ it can be rejected.

D: T

E: T Spearman rho is the equivalent non-parametric test.

60.

A: T The time interval is usually taken as one year.

B: T

C: T This is similar to kappa statistic.

D: F The target population is the whole population about which information can be gathered - usually by means of a census.

E: T This is based on the Present State Examination and gives a level of caseness, that is the subject meets diagnostic criteria for the disorder.

61.

A: T Such as looking at a psychiatric population, one subsample of which is on medication, the other, not.

B: F It is used to assess 2 variables.

C: F This is where the subjects are selected randomly prior to the investigation.

D: F This is a type of sampling called purposive sampling.

E: T For example the number of ECT treatments. In this case the dependent variable would be mood change.

PHENOMENOLOLGY

62. **The oneroid state**
    A: occurs in sleep
    B: results in vivid imagery like a waking dream
    C: when prolonged, is called a twilight state
    D: is usually induced by cannabis
    E: is associated with clouding of consciousness

63. **In monosymptomatic hypochondriacal psychosis**
    A: deterioration of personality usually occurs
    B: over-valued ideas are the main feature
    C: thioridazine is the treatment of choice
    D: can be regarded as a kind of depression
    E: delusional parasitosis is common

64. **The 'gaslight phenomenon' is**
    A: the tendency to make visual misinterpretations in conditions of poor illumination
    B: a form of *folie a deux*
    C: a form of hysterical psychosis
    D: a sub-acute encephalopathy caused by carbon monoxide
    E: the induction by deception, of what appears to be mental illness in another individual, for personal gain.

62.
A: **F**
B: **T** Mayer-Gross described psychotic states in which a dream-like change of conscoiusness was present.
C: **T**
D: **F** Usually causes alterations of affect, depersonalisation, confusion or occasionally acute paranoid reactions.
E: **T** There may be marked perplexity with the impression of disorientation.

63.
A: **F** This syndrome, described by Munro (*Brit J Hosp Med*, 1980; p34-7), is a variant of the paranoid states which are characteristically late in onset and do not lead to personality deterioration. Other examples include erotomania, litigious paranoia and some cases of dysmorphophobia.
B: **F** May begin as an overvalued idea but belief must be of delusional intensity.
C: **F** Pimozide, a specifically D2 dopamine receptor blocker is said to be the treatment of choice.
D: **F** Must be distinguished from depressive delusions (including nihilistic delusions of Cotard's syndrome).
E: **T**

64.
A: **F** This applies to delirium
B: **F** *Folie a deux* is a similar phenomenon whereby two persons, most commonly mother and daughter, share the same delusional system, where only one is truly psychotic.
C: **F**
D: **F** Carbon monoxide can cause an acute and chronic encephalopathy, Korsakoff's syndrome and extrapyramidal signs.
E: **T** Described by Barton & Whitehead in 1969 after a play called 'Gaslight'.

65. Depersonalisation
A: is usually a pleasant experience
B: is usually noticed by an observer
C: is more common in female patients
D: may be mistaken for schizophrenia
E: is more common in epileptics who are depressed than those who are euthymic

66. In psychopathology
A: forced grasping and the grasp reflex describe the same phenomena
B: *mitgehen* is an extreme form of *mitmachen*
C: logoclonia describes perseveration of the last syllable of a word
D: echolalia is specific to coarse brain disease
E: automatic obedience is common in catatonia

67. In organic psychiatric nosology
A: the eyes can be opened in stupor
B: akinetic mutism is caused by mid-brain lesions
C: clouding of consciousness is invariably associated with drowsiness
D: diurnal rhythm of activity is altered with impairment of consciousness
E: recall of events seldom occurs following alteration of consciousness

65.
A: **F** The core feeling of 'unreality' is always unpleasant.
B: **F** The feeling is entirely subjective
C: **T** But there is an equal sex incidence in healthy individuals where it may occur in as many as 50%.
D: **T** Especially when in association with depression in an unsophisticated patient who cannot describe the symptoms fully.
E: **T** Especially so with psychomotor epilepsy.

66.
A: **F** Forced grasping refers to the persistent shaking of the profferred hand despite instructions not to do so, whereas the grasp reflex is the automatic grasping of anything placed in the hand.
B: **T** *Mitgehen* is the German word describing the phenomenon whereby parts of the body can be placed in odd positions with minimal pressure - *mitmachen* is the same but requires stronger pressure.
C: **T** Palilalia is the perseveration of the last word in a sentence.
D: **F** May also be found in mental retardation, early childhood, catatonia and in fatigue.
E: **T** But also occurs in some dementing conditions.

67.
A: **T** This differentiates it from coma where the eyes are shut. Eyes may be open in cases of akinetic mutism, the so-called 'coma vigil'.
B: **T** Characteristically caused by lesions of the diencephalon, especially around the third ventricle.
C: **F** Usually drowsiness is on the spectrum from wakefulness to sleep whereas clouding of consciousness is on the spectrum to coma. Such a patient may be more excitable.
D: **T** Somnolence during the day with increased activity at night (day-night reversal).
E: **T** In contrast to stupor.

68. **In perceptual disorders**
A: chloropsia is the experience of seeing things coloured green
B: macropsia can be produced by normal ocular accomodation but weak convergence
C: an illusion is a perception without an object
D: pareidolia are the occurence of vivid illusions with little effort
E: an illusion occurs when both the provoking stimulus and perception are perceived by the subject

69. **In stupor**
A: mutism is essential to the diagnosis
B: depression is found in 25% of cases
C: resolution occurs spontaneously in 10%
D: the mortality is 30%
E: mild cases have a better prognosis

70. **Synaesthesia**
A: is a kind of reflex hallucination
B: is typical of schizophrenia
C: describes the ability to hear colours
D: includes autoscopy
E: includes extracampine hallucinations

68.

A: T Xanthopsia is yellow (may occur in digoxin toxicity), erythropsia is red.

B: T Micropsia may be caused by weak accomodation and normal convergence.

C: F This is a hallucination. An illusion is a false perception of a real object/stimulus.

D: T They do not occur as a result of a change of affect but are the result of vivid imagination and fantasy.

E: F This is a functional hallucination. In an illusion, the environmental stimulus forms an indistinguishable part of the new perception.

69.

A: T Akinesis, mutism with relative preservation consciousness is the triad.

B: T Organic causes account for 20% and schizophrenia 30% (Joyston-Bechal, (1966), *Brit J Psychiat,* 112: 967-81).

C: F About one third. The majority are terminated by physical therapy (eg ECT).

D: F Not as high, more like 20%.

E: F There may be trend for severe stupor to have a better prognosis.

70.

A: T This describes the perception of a stimulus in a different sensory modality.

B: F More typical of states induced by mescaline and other hallucinogens. Can occur in normal people and schizophrenics.

C: T

D: F This is the experience of seeing oneself and occurs in normal subjects, especially when tired, depersonalisation, epilepsy with parieto-occipital lesions, hysteria and schizophrenia.

E: F This is a hallucination outside the sensory field, for example seeing a person behind one's back.

SCHIZOPHRENIA

71. **A first episode of schizophrenia is more likely to occur**
A: after a positive life event
B: after life events in the preceding 6 months
C: at an earlier age in women
D: in the summer
E: if a person's mother is schizophrenic rather than their father

72. **First rank symptoms of schizophrenia**
A: rarely occur in mania
B: form the basis of PSE criteria for schizophrenia
C: form the basis of DSMIII criteria for schizophrenia
D: are concordant in twins, concordant for schizophrenia
E: predict a poor outcome

73. **In a twenty-year-old man, the following support a diagnosis of schizophrenia:**
A: thought insertion
B: depressive ideas
C: thought withdrawal
D: second person auditory hallucinations commenting on the person's actions
E: delusional mood

71.
A: T
B: F Life events (positive and negative) in the preceding 3 months seem to be most important. In depression the period is longer and events involving loss are more relevant.
C: F Earlier in men.
D: T
E: F The risk is equal.

72.
A: F Up to 30% in some studies.
B: T The so-called nuclear syndrome.
C: F These are based on the presence of delusions and hallucinations, social deterioration and a history of 6 months or longer. This has been termed neo-Kraepelinian as it conforms to Kraepelin's criteria for schizophrenia with its deteriorating course.
D: F The symptoms have low heritability.
E: F They are poor predictors of course. Their virtue lies in their reliability and the fact that they differ from normal phenomena.

73.
A: T
B: F Depressive symptoms are common but not diagnostic.
C: T
D: F Third person auditory hallucinations. A,C and E are examples of Schneiderian first rank symptoms (see previous question).
E: T

74. **Thought disorder in schizophrenia**
    A: was one of Bleuler's primary symptoms
    B: can be distinguished from mania by the presence of clang associations in the latter
    C: includes desultory thinking
    D: was not noted by Kraepelin
    E: shows increased redundancy

75. **The following are features of schizophrenic thought disorder:**
    A: delusional misinterpretation
    B: language disorder
    C: word finding difficulties
    D: drivelling
    E: confabulation

76. **Support for a viral aetiology of schizophrenia comes from**
    A: the long-term effects of encephalitis lethargica
    B: the increased incidence of schizophrenia in monozygotic twins compared to dizygotic
    C: the observation that schizophrenia is commoner in people born in the winter months
    D: the finding of a transmissible agent in the CSF of some schizophrenics
    E: transmission of the disease within a tribe in New Guinea by eating the brains of dead relatives

74.

A: **T** Loosening of associations, along with ambivalence, autism and loss of affect (the 4 A's).

B: **F** In mania, thought disorder includes typically, clang associations, punning and flight of ideas. These can be found in schizophrenia but tend to be more idiosyncratic and less humourous.

C: **F** Found in depression. Grammar and syntax are preserved.

D: **F** Derailment was a term coined by him.

E: **F** Reduced. This is tested by the Cloze procedure whereby words are deleted at regular intervals from a sentence and the understandability of it assessed. Schizophrenics are less understandable because they have less redundancy.

75.

A: **F** Delusions and hallucinations are not classed as examples of thought disorder.

B: **T** Spoken or written language.

C: **F** Language disorder may be difficult to distinguish from aphasia; word finding difficulties suggest the latter.

D: **T** One thought sliding into another.

E: **F** This refers to the non-deliberate fabrication of false memories due to a severe deficit in memory. May have a grandiose, wish fulfilling quality.

76.

A: **T** This epidemic produced a variant of Parkinson's disease characterised by behavioural abnormalities and oculogyric crises. Psychotic symptoms are also a feature.

B: **F** Difficult to explain by infection since all twins share the same intrauterine and to an extent, extrauterine environment.

C: **T** The excess of schizophrenia in winter births has been found in many studies in both northern and southern hemispheres. It is possible that this is due to increase liability to infection in the perinatal period.

D: **F** This has never been demonstrated.

E: **F** This refers to the transmission of virus particles responsible for the dementing illness, Kuru.

77. **The incidence of schizophrenia is higher in**
    A: Norwegian migrants to America compared to the indigenous population
    B: Northern Ireland compared to Southern Ireland
    C: Hutterites compared to manic depression
    D: persons with Down's syndrome compared to other causes of mental handicap
    E: families with elderly fathers

78. **A genetic aetiology for schizophrenia is supported by**
    A: increased concordance between dizygotic twins compared to siblings
    B: increased concordance between same sexed twins compared different sexed
    C: a concordance rate of < 50% in some series of monozygotic twins
    D: probandwise concordance being > pairwise
    E: an excess of winter births of schizophrenics

79. **The following features are associated with suicide in schizophrenics:**
    A: male sex
    B: increased age
    C: acute illness
    D: feelings of hopelessness
    E: high premorbid educational achievement

77.

A: **T** Probably due to selection factors amongst those who chose to emigrate rather than the stress of immigration. But this depends on the reasons for migration such as that forced by persecution and also the strictness of migration laws.

B: **F** Increased in Southern Ireland.

C: **F** This is an anabaptist religious community in North America, which has a higher incidence of manic depression than schizophrenia, thought to be due to genetic factors and consanguinous marriages.

D: **F**

E: **T** Could be due to schizoid personality traits leading to late marriage or perhaps increased genetic mutation in ageing sperm.

78.

A: **F** They have the same status as relatives.

B: **F** Unless a specific X-linked condition is being proposed.

C: **T** Though environmental factors must also be relevant.

D: **F** Probandwise is just a method of calculating concordance by counting each member of a twin pair, which gives a higher concordance than when pairs are counted together (pairwise).

E: **F** Supports an infective aetiology.

79.

A: **T** Plus, recent inpatient discharge and unemployment.

B: **F** Relatively young schizophrenics are more likely to kill themselves.

C: **F** Chronic illness with many relapses and remissions.

D: **T** Plus depression, feelings of inadequacy, non-delusional high expectations of themselves.

E: **T** As is living alone.

80. Expressed emotion (EE)
- A: arose out of the observation that schizophrenic patients were more liable to relapse when they were discharged to their families
- B: is derived from assessments of family interaction
- C: takes account of positive comments as well as negative
- D: if high, may result in a relapse rate of over 90% if the patient is not on neuroleptics
- E: affects depressed patients at a higher threshold

81. The prognosis of schizophrenia
- A: is improved if the patient is married
- B: is poorer in countries with poor psychiatric facilities
- C: is not influenced by EE in non-western countries
- D: is better if onset includes perplexity
- E: depends on premorbid functioning

82. Catatonia is associated with the following:
- A: Kahlbaum
- B: catalepsy
- C: cataplexy
- D: occasionally lethal cases
- C: automatism

80.

A: **T** As compared with those discharged to hostels/bedsits

B: **F** EE is assessed from the Camberwell Family Interview which is administered to the single most relevant relative. Family interaction may then be inferred from this.

C: **T** EE consists of critical comments, overinvolvement, hostility. positive remarks and warmth. So far only the 'negative' aspects have been looked at with regard to relapse of schizophrenia.

D: **T** 92%. The figure is 53% if the patient is on neuroleptic drugs at the same level of contact with relatives.

E: **F** At a lower threshold. EE is not specific to schizophrenia.

81.

A: **T** Probably reflects the absence of schizoid traits.

B: **F** A W.H.O. study has recently confirmed that prognosis is better in underdeveloped countries.

C: **F** EE has been found to exert similar effects in Chandigarh, India.

D: **T**

E: **T** Strauss and Carpenter ((1974), *Arch Gen Psychiat,* 30: 429.) found that premorbid social adjustment was the best predictor of post-illness functioning.

82.

A: **T** Described by him in 1874

B: **T** The maintenance of any posture in which the patient is placed.

C: **F** Part of the narcolepsy complex. It refers to sudden loss of muscle tone with the preservation of consciousness.

D: **T** Stauder's lethal catatonia. May be a viral encephalitis.

E: **F** This is a kind of psychomotor seizure. Automatic obedience is a catatonic sign.

AFFECTIVE DISORDER

83. **The following are believed to be biological markers for depression:**
    A: shortened REM latency
    B: suppression of cortisol secretion following dexamethasone
    C: blunted TSH response to TRH
    D: HLA-B8
    E: early morning wakening

84. **The diagnosis of primary mania is unlikely if**
    A: the patient is over 70
    B: the patient has depressive ideation
    C: a course of antidepressants was started 3 days previously
    D: the patient has evidence of early dementia
    E: there is no previous history of affective disorder

85. **Deliberate self poisoning**
    A: is frequently regarded by the patient as an attempt to influence his or her circumstances
    B: has a recurrence rate of 10% in one year
    C: is associated with an increased risk in the unemployed
    D: is associated with a major depressive episode in <5% of patients
    E: accounts for 80% of all cases of deliberate self harm

83.
A: T This is the period between going to sleep and the first period of REM sleep. Antidepressants increase REM latency.
B: F Non-suppression is a marker.
C: T This does not seem to be related to dexamethasone non-suppression.
D: F Genetic evidence has come from recent linkage studies which show a possible abnormality of the X chromosome in some pedigrees.
E: F Not a marker but sometimes referred to as a 'biological symptom' of depression.

84.
A: T Does occur rarely, but differential diagnosis in this age group includes early dementia, especially frontal lobe syndrome and toxic confusional state.
B: F Frequently mixed with manic symptoms.
C: F Too early. Commonly takes up to 10 days for antidepressants to precipitate mania.
D: F (see answer A) According to Foulds' hierarchy, one would not make the diagnosis of a functional illness in the presence of an organic condition.
E: T

85.
A: F This motivation is however frequently inferred by close relatives.
B: T
C: T Up to 5 times in some studies. However, as unemployment becomes more 'normal' its strength as a risk factor lessens.
D: F Probably around 10%. Alcoholism is common in males (25%) and is present in 5-10% of females.
E: F 90% or more. Most commonly, prescribed hypnotic drugs.

86. Studies of CSF in depression indicate
A: reduced levels of 5-hydroxyindole acetic acid (5-HIAA)
B: reduced levels of 5-HIAA in mania
C: low 5-HIAA after clinical recovery
D: elevated zinc levels
E: increased 5-hydroxytryptamine (5-HT) turnover in the brain

87. In affective disorder
A: 60% of bipolar cases begin before the age of 50
B: an untreated bipolar episode would have an average duration of 2 years
C: the length of remission between manic episodes does not alter significantly after the third episode
D: the average onset of a bipolar disorder is about the age of 30
E: the average onset of a unipolar illness is about the age of 20

88. In neuro-endocrine studies of affective disorder
A: non-suppression to the dexamethasone suppression test occurs in 90% of severe depressives
B: a blunted TRH response to TSH may be found
C: non-supression to the DST may be affected by concurrent medication
D: non-supression to the DST may predict response to medication
E: there is an increased release of growth hormone in response to clonidine

89. The following may cause a reduction in tricyclic antidepressant levels:
A: glutethimide
B: coumarols
C: orphenadrine
D: methaqualone
E: chlorpromazine

89.

A: **T**   Liver enzyme induction with barbiturates, glutethimide, rifampicin, phenytoin and methaqualone resulting in reduced tricyclic levels.

C: **T**

D: **F**

E: **F**   Although lower levels have been found in post-mortem brains of suicides.

87.

A: **F**   Approximately 90% occur before the age of 50.

B: **F**   The average duration is 13 months.

C: **T**

D: **T**   The earlier the onset, the poorer the prognosis. Note also that relatives of bipolar patients have a greater chance of developing an affective disorder (uni or bipolar) than relatives of unipolar patients.

E: **F**   This varies widely and has no upper or lower age limit.

88.

A: **F**   Closer to 60%.

B: **F**   Read each question carefully! It is the TSH response to TRH.

C: **T**   As well as age, weight, sleep deprivation and activity.

D: **T**   Remains controversial.

E: **F**   There is a blunted GH response to clonidine.

89.

A: **T**   Liver enzyme induction with barbiturates, glutethimide, rifampicin, phenytoin and methaqualone resulting in reduced tricyclic levels.

B: **F**

C: **F**

D: **T**

E: **F**   May increase levels.

90. The following are scales used for the assessment of depression:
A: Montgomery and Asberg
B: Hamilton
C: Zung
D: Wakefield
E: Von Zerssens

91. The following are classifications of affective disorder in ICD9:
A: schizo-affective disorder
B: non-organic psychoses excitative type
C: affective personality disorder
D: cyclothymic disorder
E: adjustment disorder with depressed mood

92. The following apply to suicide:
A: incidence is increasing in old age
B: females commit suicide more often than males
C: seasonal variation is more marked in males
D: the frequency is higher in urban than in rural areas
E: incidence is lowest in social class I

90.
A: T   10 items selected for frequency of occurence.
B: T   17 item scale covering most common symptoms.
C: T   Zung self-rating depression scale.
D: T   Consists of 12 items in four grades. Self assessment scale.
E: T   This is an adjective checklist. Also of proven value are visual analogue scales and the Beck Depression Index.

91.
A: F   Note the word 'disorder' which is used frequently in DSMIII and sparingly in ICD9. Useful to distinguish and remember: In ICD9 this comes under schizophrenia whereas in DSMIII it is based among the major affective disorders.
B: T   The word 'type' occurs regularly in ICD9. Note that ICD10 will be out soon and will probably include a multi-axial classifcation like DSMIII.
C: T   Disorder is used in relation to personality in ICD9.
D: F   This is a DSMIII classification under other specific affective disorders and classed with dysthymic disorder.
E: F   In ICD9 it is adjustment reaction with brief or prolonged depressive reaction.

92.
A: F   If anything it is decreasing.
B: F   Males more common than females in all age groups. Parasuicide is considerably more common in females. Males tend to choose more aggressive means such as hanging and shooting.
C: F   More marked in females.
D: T
E: F   Lowest in social class II.

93. **The amine hypothesis of affective disorder is supported by**
A: low concentrations of 5HIAA in the CSF of depressed
      patients
B: decreased acetylcholine levels in the brain
C: the antidepressant action of tryptophan
D: increased incidence of depression in the winter months
      in certain individuals
E: the antidepressant action of phenelzine

94. **The following drugs may be prescribed for a depressed man 2
months after a myocardial infarction:**
A: amitriptyline
B: lofepramine
C: doxepin
D: mianserin
E: trimipramine

93.
A: T Also decreased levels of 5HT and 5HIAA in the raphe nuclei of post mortem brains of suicide victims.
B: F Related to Alzheimer's Disease.
C: T A precursor of 5HT.
D: T Possibly related to melatonin effects.
E: T A monoamine oxidase inhibitor

94.
A: F This has more marked anticholinergic and cardiac side effects and should be avoided in ischaemic heart disease.
B: T
C: T
D: T Lofepramine, doxepin, dothiepin and mianserin all have less cardiac side effects but should still be used cautiously.
E: F As with amitriptyline, these may cause arrhythmias and heart block.

CHILD PSYCHIATRY/MENTAL HANDICAP

95. The following are true of childhood autism:
   A: symptoms tend to begin around the third year of life
   B: the word autism originally referred to abnormalities of speech
   C: boys are affected more than girls
   D: an abnormal reaction to sound is common
   E: a better prognosis is favoured by a high I.Q.

96. Child sex abuse
   A: may happen in up to 10% of families
   B: with father daughter incest, occurs in 1% of families
   C: affects boys in 10% of cases
   D: by a stranger, accounts for a third of all cases
   E: can be detected by physical examination in about 15% of cases

97. The clinical features of Down's syndrome include:
   A: mouth breathing
   B: transverse palmar crease in 75%
   C: eczema
   D: decreased MCV (mean red cell volume)
   E: absence of any pattern on the hallucal area of the sole

98. Down's syndrome with a translocated chromosome
   A: is always inherited from one parent
   B: may be related to advancing paternal age
   C: where a parent is a 21/21 translocation chromosome carrier all children will be affected
   D: accounts for 10% of Down's syndrome children
   E: the risk is lower where the father is the carrier

95.

A: F Symptoms almost always begin before the age of three and most experts say they have been present since birth.

B: F The word (coined by Bleuler) was used originally by Kanner to describe a disturbance of affective contact.

C: T The exact sex incidence is between 2.75:1 and 4.5:1 with males predominating.

D: T There is often either an excessive response to sounds or no response (in which case deafness is in the differential diagnosis).

E: T In one study 15% of patients had improved at follow-up; 25% had a modest improvement but were still handicapped and 60% had experienced some lessening of the handicaps. A high I.Q. favoured a good prognosis.

96.

A: T More common than previously thought but precise incidence difficult to calculate.

B: T Father and step-father/daughter incest is by far the most common.

C: F 20-40%

D: F Less common, around 10-15%

E: T Genital and rectal injury or venereal disease.

97.

A: T Leads to an increased risk of upper respiratory tract infections.

B: F 30-40%.

C: F Occurs in phenylketonuria.

D: F MCV is raised in many non-anaemic subjects.

E: T In 50%.

98.

A: F It is unusual but both may be carriers. It is possible to deduce this answer from the other questions.

B: T Advancing paternal age may be a significant factor in the 21/22 translocation group.

C: T This is fortunately rare but when present all children are affected.

D: F Probably less than 2% are genetically transmitted.

E: T

99. In sex chromosomal abnormalities
A: the degree of physical and mental handicap is related to the number of extra X chromosomes
B: incidence is independent of maternal age
C: there is an inverse ratio between the number of X chromosomes and the ridge count in dermatoglyphics
D: amniocentesis is less reliable in a multiple pregnancy
E: approximately 10% of people with an additional X chromosome are mosaics

100. In child psychiatric referral
A: a high proportion of G.P. referrals are for psychosomatic problems
B: the referral rate differs significantly between schools
C: social disadvantage is not associated
D: the emotional stability of the father is an influential factor
E: the majority of eneuretics have been referred by the age of 10

101. Children with failure to thrive and growth retardation
A: are delayed in their cognitive development
B: have a history of low birth weight
C: have an underlying organic condition in approximately 50%
D: should be assessed using cross-sectional data
E: may occasionally arise from maternal rejection

102. Childhood obesity is associated with
A: de Lange syndrome
B: Laurence-Moon-Biedel syndrome
C: Prader Willi syndrome
D: tuberose sclerosis
E: lower social class

103. In faecal soiling
A: soiling rarely occurs at night
B: there is an equal incidence in boys and girls
C: retention with overflow occurs in a small number of cases
D: prognosis is worse when associated with behavioural problems
E: history of anal fissure is rare

99.
A: T The effect is less marked for females.
B: T
C: T
D: T In a multiple pregnancy samples should be obtained from each amniotic sac with the aid of ultrasound.
E: F About one third are mosaics.

100.
A: F These would generally be referred to a paediatrician.
B: T May be related to school circumstances.
C: F
D: F Epidemiological research has shown that the mother's emotional stability affects GP's readiness to refer, but not the father's.
E: F The majority never reach a clinic.

101.
A: T
B: T
C: F Approximately one third have an organic component.
D: F Serial height and weight data should be used.
E: F This is more than an occasional feature but should not be assumed.

102.
A: F Dwarfism, skeletal abnormalities and severe mental retardation.
B: T Mental retardation and polydactyly.
C: T Hypogonadism, ataxia and diabetes.
D: F Epilepsy, abnormal skin pigmentation and usually mental retardation.
E: T

103.
A: T When it does it is associated with a poor prognosis.
B: F Occurs in boys three times more often.
C: F This may occur in up to three quarter of cases.
D: T
E: F This is common and important to exclude.

104. In the treatment of enuresis with a bell and pad
A: response may take up to the second month of treatment
B: in the mentally retarded response may take up to six months
C: response may be related to maternal anxiety
D: response may be related to the age of the child
E: a cure is 7 nights of continuous dryness

105. Enuresis is associated with
A: temper tantrums
B: fire-setting
C: cruelty to animals
D: a more retiring nature
E: a disturbance in urinary circadian rhythm

106. School refusal
A: is commonest at 9 years of age
B: may occur after a respiratory tract infection
C: in older children may have a more insidious onset
D: is less associated with neurotic traits than truancy
E: has a worse prognosis in older children

107. Nocturnal enuresis
A: occurs during REM sleep
B: is not associated with encopresis
C: occurs in 7% of children at age 7
D: may be treated using the pad and bell technique, an example of operant conditioning
E: treatment with imipramine is superior to amitriptyline

104.
A: T
B: T
C: T
D: F
E: F A cure is defined as 14 nights of continuous dryness.

105.
A: F
B: F
C: F
D: T
E: F Enuretics show the cycle whereby the production of urine is reduced to one third of its day time level at night.

106.
A: F Most common at age 5 (starting school), 7 (change to junior school) and 11, (starting secondary school). Slightly more common in boys.
B: T Many minor life events may precipitate it.
C: T
D: F Is more associated with neurotic traits. These may persist into adult life resulting in a higher incidence of psychiatric disorders especially agoraphobia.
E: T Often a family approach combined with legal enforcement of the child attending school is most effective.

107.
A: F Usually in slow wave sleep as do night terrors.
B: F Beware the double negative!
C: F 7% of *boys* at age 7. Male:female ratio is approx 3:1.
D: F Classical conditioning.
E: F Both are effective. Mechanism unclear, unrelated to effect on mood. 85% response but high relapse rate on stopping drug, despite duration of treatment.

108. In the Isle of Wight child psychiatry epidemiology study
- A: the prevalence of psychiatric disorder in boys was twice that in girls
- B: the prevalence of psychiatric disorder increased as intelligence decreased
- C: uncomplicated epilepsy was not a significant risk factor
- D: on follow-up 4 years later over half were still handicapped by their problems
- E: the subsequent inner London survey found broadly similar rates

109. Conduct disorder
- A: forms the largest single group of psychiatric disorders in older children
- B: was associated with an IQ slightly below average in girls in the Isle of Wight study
- C: is strongly associated with educational retardation
- D: runs a 3 to 5 year course
- E: if socialized, carries a better prognosis

110. Physical abuse in children
- A: occurs in 1:1000 children under 4
- B: results in 25% being intellectually damaged
- C: also affects 70% of the siblings of the originally identified battered child
- D: is more likely to occur when the child is premature
- E: is associated with unemployment in 50% of the fathers

108.
A: T
B: T
C: F Epilepsy is a risk factor. The prevalence of psychiatric disorder was 34% in children with seizures. Epilepsy with brain damage and with a temporal lobe focus carried the highest risk.
D: T
E: F The rate was double (13% vs. 6.8%)

109.
A: T 4% of Isle of Wight children. 1.1% had aggressive conduct disorder.
B: F True for boys. True for emotional disorders in girls.
C: T
D: F 50% had some form of antisocial behaviour in adulthood
E: T The best predictor of poor outcome is the extent of childhood antisocial behaviour.

110.
A: T The figure may be higher than this!
B: T Due to repeated head injuries.
C: F Closer to 20%.
D: T One of the child characteristics that has been seen most persistently as leading to increased abuse.
E: T Unemployment, social isolation and experience of abuse in the parents' own childhood are associated with an increased risk of abuse.

111. The following are associated with brain damage in a 10 year old child:
A: specific reading retardation
B: conduct disorder
C: impulsivity
D: deprived family background
E: disintegrative psychosis

112. The following are autosomal recessive conditions:
A: phenylketonuria
B: Huntington's disease
C: Hunter's syndrome
D: albinism
E: galactosaemia

111.

A: T   The Isle of Wight study showed that the brain damaged population had an increased incidence of specific reading retardation, below average I.Q., and physical handicap.

B: T   If the appropriate social stressors occur then brain damaged children are more likely to develop anti-social conduct disorder.

C: F   There was no excess of overactivity and impulsivity.

D: T   This has an additive effect with social disadvantage more common among disturbed brain injured children than in brain injured children without psychiatric disturbance.

E: T   Disintegrative psychosis, autism and confusional states.

112.

A: T

B: F   Autosomal dominant.

C: F   X-linked recessive - not to be confused with Hurler's syndrome, which is autosomal recessive and where the mental and physical deterioration is more rapid.

D: T

E: T

NEUROSES

113. In obsessive compulsive neurosis
- A: resistance is an essential component of the compulsion
- B: is clearly linked to harsh toilet training in infancy
- C: obsessive-compulsive symptoms may occur as a result of encephalitis lethargica
- D: prevalence in the general population is about 1%
- E: clomipramine is only successful when depressive elements are present

114. Anxiety neurosis is
- A: the second commonest form of neurosis in the Western World
- B: said to occur in 15% of first degree relatives of affected subjects
- C: the reason behind nearly 30% of general practice consultations
- D: a cause of bilateral coarse intention tremor
- E: more associated with somatisation in more intelligent patients

115. Patients with panic disorder
- A: may have attacks induced by lactate infusions
- B: have a 25% chance of having a similarly affected first degree relative
- C: often have mitral valve prolapse
- D: respond to high doses of imipramine
- E: may be schizophrenic

113.

A: F Although originally thought to be an essential component, resistance is more directed against the repetition of the action, and not the action itself. It is not seen in chronic patients, post-leucotomy or as part of childhood rituals.

B: F Although psycho-analytic theory links obsessive compulsive neurosis to anal fixation there is little supporting evidence.

C: T

D: F It is very rare, approximately 0.05%.

E: F This is a controversial issue but the wording 'only successful' should alert the candidate that it is unlikely to be true.

114.

A: F It is the commonest form, thought to affect 2-5% of the population.

B: T

C: T And just under 10% of psychiatric outpatient referrals.

D: T Intention tremor as in performance anxiety. Must be distinguished from thyrotoxicosis and alcoholic withdrawal 'shakes'.

E: F

115.

A: T Not a specific test. Not all patients respond in this way but are more likely to than normals.

B: T

C: F Most patients with mitral valve prolapse do not have panic attacks though they are at a higher risk of cardiac arrhythmias than the general population.

D: F Said to respond specifically to low doses. Also responds to new benzodiazepine, alprazolam.

E: T Patients with schizophrenia may also suffer from anxiety.

116. Munchausen syndrome
A: is a disorder which affects males predominantly
B: most commonly involves neurological symptoms
C: has a mean age of presentation of 25 years
D: is frequently a manifestation of depression
E: is best managed by blacklisting the patient

117. With regard to conversion hysteria:
A: 'belle indifference' is diagnostic
B: Plato was first to describe hysteria as a disease of the mind
C: hysterical personalities tend to have high 'E' scores on the Eysenck Personality Inventory
D: 50% of patients with hysteria have previous hysterical personalities
E: lowering of peripheral receptor sensitivity has been found in patients with hysterical anaesthesia

118. The following statements apply to phobias:
A: thassophobia is the fear of sitting idle
B: animal phobias have an equal sex incidence
C: a strong genetic component has been identified
D: a large proportion of social phobics have a timid and shy pre-morbid personality
E: desensitisation in fantasy is most successful when free-floating anxiety is present

116.

A: F 50% are male.

B: F Abdominal symptoms and haemoptysis are the most common

C: F 36 is the mean age.

D: F A minority have treatable depression the remainder have severe personality difficulties.

E: F This helps the hospital but does little for the individual.

117.

A: F Neither diagnostic nor common in hysterics. Over dramatic presentation or apparent indifference to disability are best described in terms of abnormal illness behaviour (Pilowsky). This gets away from the problem of making strict 'organic' or 'functional' judgements. Patients often have a history of 'genuine' disability or develop it later, as Eliot Slater showed in his follow-up study of hysterics seen at the National Hospital, Queen Square.

B: F Sydenham was, in 1681.

C: T

D: F The figure is 12-21%.

E: T

118.

A: T A common complaint amongst exam candidates!

B: F Much commoner in women.

C: F Little evidence for this at present. In contrast to blood-injury phobia which has a strong genetic component. May be qualitatively different since the fainting response is parasympathetic in contrast to the exaggerated sympathetic response to other phobic stimuli.

D: T

E: F Flooding is the treatment of choice here - desensitisation is better where free-floating anxiety is absent.

119. In hypochondriasis
A: symptoms usually occur in the absence of other psychiatric conditions
B: unilateral symptoms affect mainly the left side
C: the patient rarely wishes to know about the underlying disorder
D: the female to male ratio is 3:1 in the primary form
E: the incidence is highest in middle age

120. Patients with onset of neurosis starting in later life, compared to those with chronic neurosis, are more likely to
A: have low income
B: be late in birth order
C: have had poor relationships with their parents
D: have physical disability
E: be lonely

121. The Ganser syndrome
A: occurs in clear consciousness
B: includes hallucinations
C: may herald schizophrenia
D: is characterised by *vorbeireden*
E: may be more common than originally thought

119.
A: **F** Rarely - often occurs in a setting of depression, (especially in non-European cultures such as Asians) obsessional disorders as well as paranoid states and schizophrenia.
B: **T**
C: **F** This is characteristic of somatisation disorder (*syn* Briquet's hysteria). In hypochondriasis, the patient usually inquires about the underlying disease though fails to be reassured.
D: **F** Sex incidence is equal.
E: **F** More common in the old and the young.

120.
A: **T**
B: **F** This applies to chronic neurosis.
C: **F** Mainly those with chronic neurosis.
D: **T**
E: **T** There is evidence that neurotic disorders in early life tend to lessen with age but that late onset neurosis is a distinct entity resulting from severe stress and resulting in extreme disability.

121.
A: **F** S.J.M. Ganser described 3 prisoners with this 'peculiar hysterical state', in 1898. Changeable clouding of consciousness is one of its characteristics.
B: **T**
C: **T** Or epileptic phenomena or dementia.
D: **T** Approximate answers eg. How many legs has a donkey? Answer - five. This indicates understanding of the question and the correct reply.
E: **F** If anything it is rarer but exists in textbooks and exam MCQs!

122. The hyperventilation syndrome
A: is commonest in young women
B: causes headache
C: has a diagnostic test
D: can cause a decrease in cerebral blood flow of up to 10%
E: may exaggerate cerebral dysrhythmias in epileptics

123. In general practice
A: 40% of patients present with emotional disorders
B: emotional disturbance occurs most commonly in adolescent females
C: 10% of psychiatric disorders are referred to hospital
D: accuracy of detection of psychiatric disorder is increased by the doctor's readiness to make a psychiatric assessment
E: women are more likely to be referred to hospital

122.
A: T In up to 29% of young women referred to neurologists.
B: T Also, paraesthesia, nausea, dyspnoea, palpitations and visual disturbance.
C: T If three minutes overbreathing induces similar symptoms the diagnosis can be made.
D: F Four minutes overbreathing results in a 40% decrease in cerebral blood flow.
E: T Hyperventilation is used to provoke dysrhythmias in routine EEG recording.

123.
A: F Approximately 15% present with emotional disorders. 40% present with a combination of physical and emotional disorder.
B: F Most commonly in middle aged women.
C: F 5.5% of all diagnoses are referred for psychiatric assessment.
D: F A sympathetic bias towards psychiatric conditions does not improve accuracy - that is the doctor is more likely to diagnose a psychiatric disorder even when one is not present. Higher training and higher scores on knowledge of clinical medicine and positive self-regard do improve accuracy.
E: F Men are more likely to be referred than women - younger subjects more likely than older.

OLD AGE PSYCHIATRY

124. Delirium in the elderly
A: has a prevalence of 10%, regardless of the population studied
B: fluctuates according to the time of day, being worse in the morning
C: is alleviated by anticholinergic drugs
D: does not produce changes in affect
E: should be treated in a darkened room

125. The following scales may be used to measure cognitive impairment in the elderly:
A: The Mental Test Score
B: The Stockton Geriatric Rating Scale
C: The Psychogeriatric Dependency Rating Scale
D: The Mini-Mental State
E: The Geriatric Mental State

126. Late paraphrenia
A: is probably a form of schizophrenia
B: occurs most often in elderly men
C: deafness is a frequent accompaniment
D: premorbid personality is likely to be abnormal
E: has a higher incidence with lower social class

124.

A: **F** Prevalence varies enormously, from 8% of psychiatric patients to 80% in a geriatric medical unit.

B: **F** Fluctuation is common but the patient is characteristically worse at night.

C: **F** The elderly are particularly sensitive to the adverse cognitive effects of these drugs.

D: **F** Mood tends to be labile with sudden changes from a dazed state to extreme paranoia or excitement.

E: **F** The opposite. Studies have shown improvement in units with, as against those without, windows.

125.

A: **T** Originally developed to assess memory and correlated with post-mortem changes.

B: **F** Measures behavioural disturbance. Not a reference to the late Lord Stockton.

C: **F** This measures a variety of functions including orientation but overall is a measure 'dependency' of a patient and not cognition.

D: **T** Short and widely used screening test.

E: **T** Although a schedule to assess symptoms, it does have a section on cognition.

126.

A: **T**

B: **F** Characteristically elderly single women are affected.

C: **T**

D: **T** A schizoid personality is often found.

E: **T**

127. With regard to the population over 65 in England and Wales:
A: there was a 40% rise from 1959 to 1981
B: the over-85's increased by 50% in the same period
C: they represent 15% of the total population
D: about 6% suffer from dementia
E: 28% live alone

128. The following may occur in Alzheimer's disease:
A: raised prolactin levels in older patients
B: raised CSF prolactin concentrations
C: raised growth hormone levels in the morning
D: lowered TSH levels
E: reduced oestrogen stimulated neurophysin

129. It has been recommended that elderly psychiatric patients require
A: 1 bed per 1,000 for functional mental illness
B: 3 beds per 1,000 for those severely demented without physical illness
C: 10 beds per thousand for demented patients with physical illness
D: 10 day hospital places per 1,000 for those with dementia
E: the care of psychiatrists if they have both dementia and physical illness

127.
A: T About 1.6 million in total.
B: F The rise in the over-85's was 89%.
C: T
D: T Estimates vary between 5 and 6.4%. There are probably an additional 5% with mild cognitive impairment.
E: T A third of the over-65's have no living children.

128.
A: T Seen in senile dementia but not in the pre-senile form.
B: F If anything, it is reduced with cerebral atrophy.
C: T
D: F Low TSH and GH may be due to reduced hypothalamic somatostatin.
E: T May reflect reduced cholinergic activity.

129.
A: F The figure is 0.5 beds with 0.65 day hospital places per 1,000.
B: T
C: T With an additional 2 day hospital places per 1,000.
D: F Not as many. Three per 1,000 for both mild and severly demented patients without physical illness.
E: F These should primarily be the responsibility of the geriatrician.

130. **With regard to drugs in the elderly:**
    A: absorption declines
    B: a steady-state is achieved more rapidly than in younger patients
    C: mianserin is not contra-indicated in the presence of glaucoma
    D: the half-life (t½) of lithium is prolonged by 25-30%
    E: shortening of the Q-T interval on the ECG may occur with thioridazine

131. **The neuropathological appearances of Alzheimer's disease include**
    A: senile plaques especially in the medial temporal cortex
    B: neurofibrillary tangles especially in the limbic region
    C: Hirano bodies in the amygdala
    D: amyloid in conjunction with tangles
    E: granulovacuolar degeneration

132. **The following occur in normal ageing:**
    A: decrease in performance ability as measured by the WAIS (Wechsler Adult Intelligence Scale)
    B: slowing of reaction time
    C: decrease in digit recall
    D: decline in 'fluid' abilities
    E: decrease in recall for famous past events

130.

A: **T** Due to decreased gastric secretion and decreased intestinal blood flow.

B: **F** This is dependent on drug t½ - usually 5 t½'s are required for a steady state. Thus it is prolonged because the t½ is prolonged.

C: **T** Tricyclics are contra-indicated because anticholinergic pupil dilatation may precipitate acute glaucoma. Trazadone and mianserin are safe but caution is still advised.

D: **F** Often 50-100% - secondary to decreased renal clearance (not necessarily in the presence of discrete renal disease).

E: **F** Prolongation with 'T' wave inversion or sometimes arrhythmias may occur.

131.

A: **T** These are seen microscopically in the temporal cortex, amygdala and hippocampus.

B: **T** These intracellular structures appear as aggregated bundles of filaments. Seen in the hippocampus in normal ageing but especially in the neocortex with Alzheimer's disease (AD).

C: **F** The hippocampus. They are eosinophilic, oval structures not specific to AD.

D: **F** Amyloid (extracellular fibrillary material) is found in cerebral vessels and plaques.

E: **T** Vacuoles in cells with a central, red staining granule. Found in the hippocampus in AD.

132.

A: **T** Performance IQ starts to fall at the age of 30 but dips markedly after age 65. Verbal IQ decreases only slightly from age 30, dipping at the same time as performance.

B: **T** Reaction time falls by 20% in 60 year-olds compared to 20 year-olds,

C: **F** Not if simple recall but true for complicated recall (ie, repeating digits in reverse order)

D: **T** Fluid abilities include flexible and novel reasoning capacity (nothing to do with the urinary system!). This is in contrast to well learned skills which don't deteriorate.

E: **F**

ORGANIC PSYCHIATRY

133. In General Paralysis of the Insane
   A: changes in personality usually precede cognitive deficits
   B: the grandiose form is the commonest type
   C: pupillary abnormalities occur in 90%
   D: tremor is seldom seen
   E: serological tests (WR and VDRL) may be negative in 25% of cases

134. Huntington's disease
   A: does not begin over the age of 60
   B: may not include chorea
   C: may commonly include schizophrenic symptoms
   D: often presents with memory disorder
   E: characteristically causes isolated caudate atrophy

135. Mental symptoms in patients with cerebral tumours
   A: are seen early in 50% of cases
   B: are especially common when they are situated in the anterior and posterior corpus callosum
   C: include disturbance of consciousness more commonly when the lesion is frontal rather than occipital
   D: are more common in slowly growing tumours
   E: accompany meningiomas more than other types of neoplasms

133.
A: T
B: F This used to be the case until the 19th century but no longer.
C: F The pupillary abnormalities including Argyll Robertson pupils (small, irregular, unequal pupils which respond to accomodation but not light) occur in about two thirds of cases.
D: F A common early sign also present in two thirds of cases.
E: F They may be negative in only 10% of cases.

134.
A: F May be misdiagnosed as 'senile chorea'. Onset is usually between 25-50 years.
B: T Especially in juvenile onset cases (Westphal variant) where rigidity predominates.
C: F Can occur but affective symptoms are more common.
D: F Surprisingly rare. This parallels the neuropathology where limbic structures are spared.
E: F Caudate atrophy is characteristic but is usually accompanied by frontal lobe atrophy.

135.
A: F Overall 15% - more with frontal and temporal tumours, less in infratentorial and occipital.
B: T Up to 90% have mental symptoms, compared to about 50% of tumours of the middle part of the callosum.
C: F
D: F More common with malignant fast growing tumours.
E: T 30% have associated mental symptoms compared to 15% overall.

136. The following are examples of sub-cortical dementia:
A: Steele-Richardson syndrome
B: Korsakoff's syndrome
C: Huntington's chorea
D: Alzheimer's disease
E: Pick's disease

137. Gilles de la Tourette syndrome
A: usually has an onset after puberty
B: includes the involuntary whispering of obscenities
C: is commonly associated with non-specific neurological signs and EEG abnormalities
D: may be successfully treated with haloperidol
E: is associated with compulsions

138. The Kluver-Bucy syndrome
A: results from complete ablation of the left temporal lobe
B: includes constructional apraxia
C: causes loss of aggressiveness
D: includes hypersexuality
E: includes oral tendencies

136.

A: T This is an extrapyramidal syndrome similar to Parkinson's disease but with characteristic abnormalities of conjugate gaze, especially in the vertical plane.

B: F This is an amnestic syndrome with loss of short-term memory but other cognitive functions remain more or less intact.

C: T

D: F The most common cortical dementia. Subcortical dementia implies apathy, slowness, lack of initiative and some memory disturbance. 'Cortical' dementia implies aphasia, apraxia and agnosia as well as amnesia.

E: F A cortical dementia with a predeliction for the frontal (and temporal) lobes.

137.

A: F Onset is usually before the age of sixteen.

B: F It includes coprolalia, the involuntary shouting of obscenities.

C: T

D: T Or other butyrophenones.

E: T

138.

A: F Results from bilateral ablation of the amygdala, uncus and parts of the hippocampus (parts of the temporal lobe). This may follow head injury or herpes simplex encephalitis.

B: F Includes visual agnosia.

C: F Aggressiveness increases - there is loss of fear.

D: T

E: T The syndrome also consists of blunted affect, binge-eating, hypersexuality, hypermetamorphosis (immediate exploration of surroundings in response to stimuli), visual agnosia and amnesia.

139. Prosopagnosia
   A: is sometimes referred to as Capgras syndrome
   B: results in a failure to recognise familiar faces
   C: may be caused by a fugue state
   D: may occur in Alzheimer's disease
   E: includes failure to recognise parts of the body

140. The consequences of damage to the frontal lobes include:
   A: aphasia
   B: apathy
   C: lack of social awareness
   D: perseveration
   E: hypomania

141. Depression following a stroke
   A: is more likely to occur with left parietal lesions
   B: is more severe the nearer the lesion is to the frontal lobe
   C: correlates with the degree of intellectual impairment
   D: treatment of depression may improve cognitive function
   E: often includes delusions of self blame

139.

A: F

B: T Prosopagnosia is a rare organic syndrome caused usually by bilateral lesions of the posterior temporal/occipital lobes. It results in failure to recognise faces and characteristically affects recognition of familiar faces including immediate family and even the subjects own face. Capgras syndrome is delusional misidentification, in which the sufferer believes that those around him are mere impersonations, usually as part of a sinister plot. Organic factors may contribute to this state.

C: F But may be similar. A fugue state is a form of hysterical dissociation in which memory and orientation are seemingly lost. This invariably follows a traumatic event and is usually temporary.

D: T

E: F This is asomatognosia, a non-dominant parietal syndrome

140.

A: T Broca's area is part of the frontal lobe, damage to which results in non-fluent aphasia.

B: T Part of the frontal lobe syndrome which includes inappropriate social behaviour, perseveration, coarsening of personality and irritability. Intellect is relatively preserved.

C: T

D: T The continued response to a stimulus (eg a question or instruction) after the stimulus is withdrawn and another introduced.

E: T A bland euphoria is common but must be distinguished from hypomania which may also occur but somewhat less frequently.

141.

A: F It is more frequent and more severe with left frontal lesions.

B: T Positive correlation between the proximity to the frontal pole and severity of mood disturbance.

C: T Although this is a weaker relationship than the above (answer B).

D: T Demonstrated in a trial of nortriptyline given for 6 weeks in patients with post stroke depression.

E: F This is rare in contrast to functional disorders in this age group.

142. The following are strongly suggestive of multi-infarct dementia rather than Alzheimer's disease:
    A: memory disorder following a cerebrovascular accident
    B: a Hachinski score of two
    C: slowly progressive disease
    D: a history of hypertension
    E: a family history of dementia

143. Treatable causes of dementia include:
    A: depression
    B: mental retardation
    C: vitamin B 12 deficiency
    D: hyperthyroidism
    E: subdural haematoma

144. The epileptic aura
    A: may precede the seizure by a few hours
    B: is associated with non-specific slowing of the EEG
    C: indicates a focal structural lesion
    D: may include depersonalization
    E: is usually recalled once consciousness is regained

142.
A: T
B: F The score includes, abrupt onset, step-wise progression, signs and symptoms of cerebrovascular disease, nocturnal confusion , emotional incontinence and hypertension. A score of <4 is said to indicate a non-vascular aetiology whereas a score of >7 suggests a vascular origin. (Hachinski *et al,* (1974) *Lancet;* ii: 207-10)
C: F
D: T
E: F

143.
A: T Depressive pseudo-dementia.
B: F Dementia is an *acquired* loss of intellectual function whereas mental handicap usually describes a congenital deficit.
C: T
D: F Does not cause dementia unlike hypothyroidism which may present with progressive, global cognitive impairment as well as psychosis (myxoedema madness).
E: T May be missed in alcoholics who are prone to subdurals because of frequent falls and cirrhosis induced coagulation impairment.

144.
A: F Lasts seconds only. This must be distinguished from the much longer prodromal phase which can last hours or even days and includes alterations in mood and behaviour. The aura is not invariably followed by a full blown seizure especially if the patient is partially treated.
B: F The aura is associated with epileptic discharges (spike and wave).
C: T
D: T And other perceptual phenomena including somatic (usually gastric) sensations.
E: T

145. In epilepsy
A: gelastic epilepsy is laughing during a seizure
B: petit mal attacks last on average 1-2 minutes
C: kindling is a clinical description of an early epileptic phenomenon
D: there is an increased prevalence of psychosis
E: patients are more liable to commit crimes of violence

146. In psychosurgery
A: treatment is indicated for severe obsessional neurosis
B: amygdalotomy is effective in the treatment of uncontrolable aggressiveness
C: 80% of obsessional neurotics improve after surgery
D: two thirds of depressives treated with limbic leucotomy improve
E: limbic leucotomy interrupts limbo-striatal pathways

147. Recent research in the molecular pathology of Alzheimer's disease (AD) has shown
A: the genetic defect is on chromosome 11
B: the gene for amyloid is the same as the gene responsible for AD
C: amyloid deposits similar to those in AD have been found in primates
D: neurofibrillary tangles are more specific to AD than senile plaques
E: the core of the plaque contains inorganic aluminosilicate

145.

A: T Cursive epilepsy is running during attacks

B: F Rarely last longer than 30 seconds. Petit mal status is a rare phenomenon but does occur.

C: F This is an experimental neurophysiological term referring to the finding that repeated subthreshold stimulation may produce seizure activity in post-synaptic neurones.

D: T Those especially prone are those with temporal lobe seizures.

E: F Although there is a higher than expected prevalence of epilepsy in prisoners, the type of crime does not differ.

146.

A: F Indicated only if very severe and extensive behaviour therapy and all other treatments have failed.

B: F It is still rarely done but no proper evaluation of the technique has been made.

C: T This is claimed but again no controlled trials have been performed. 50% of patients are said to be symptom free.

D: T Again no controlled trials. Mania may respond more than depression in bipolar patients.

E: F Interrupts limbo-frontal pathways. Said to improve intractable depression.

147.

A: F There is evidence that a gene for affective disorder is on this chromosome. The gene for AD is most likely to be on the long arm of chromosome 21.

B: F They are very close on chromosome 21 but are probably not identical.

C: T This holds promise for being the first animal model for AD.

D: F They are less specific.

E: T This inorganic component and a polypeptide named A4 together make up the core of the plaque.

PERSONALITY DISORDER/FORENSIC PSYCHIATRY

148. With respect to the Mental Health Act (1983)
- A: nurse's holding power of patients already in hospital is 12 hours
- B: doctor's holding power under section 5(2) is 72 hours
- C: common law dictates that anyone can restrain a patient in an emergency
- D: compulsory admission can be applied for under section 4 for a maximum of 48 hours
- E: a treatability clause was introduced to cover the mentally handicapped

149. The category of Borderline Personality Disorder
- A: is no longer included in the Diagnostic and Statistical Manual (DSMIII) of the American Psychiatric Association
- B: is not included in the International Classification of Diseases (ICD-9)
- C: includes people previously regarded as latent schizophrenics
- D: refers to individuals on the borderline between normality and personality disorder
- E: includes chronic feelings of boredom and emptiness

150. Studies of personality have shown
- A: that extraverted and histrionic individuals are more easily sedated
- B: a strong genetic influence on obsessionality
- C: social introversion is substantially more influenced by environment than heredity
- D: people who have dependent traits are more suggestible
- E: concordance rates of MZ twins for delinquency is higher in adults compared to juveniles

148.
A: **F** The maximum duration is 6 hours under section 5(4).
B: **T**
C: **T** Under common law anyone can act in an emergency as long as the patient presents an imminent danger to himself or others.
D: **F** Section 4 runs for 72 hours.
E: **F** The treatability clause was introduced mainly for individuals with personality disorders.

149.
A: **F** Criteria include: impulsivity, unstable relationships, displays of anger, identity disturbance, affective instability, intolerance of being alone, emptiness and boredom.
B: **T** Not a popular diagnosis outside the USA. Regarded as merely a severe form of the other more established categories of personality disorder.
C: **T** An old concept encompassing schizoid individuals with a propensity to develop psychosis under stress.
D: **F** The 'borderline' is between personality disorder and psychosis.
E: **T** See above.

150.
A: **T** They have a lower threshold to sedative and hypnotic drugs.
B: **F** Note the question refers to obsessionality and not obsessional neurosis which has an appreciable genetic component.
C: **F** Introversion and extraversion even in animals, seems to be under more genetic control.
D: **T**
E: **T** Genetic factors confirmed by the Danish adoption studies.

151. Exhibitionists
A: usually masturbate at the time of exposure
B: tend to be over the age of 40 years
C: tend to be of normal intelligence
D: most reoffenders do so in the first year after conviction
E: often expose themselves to people they know

152. Section 136 of the 1983 Mental Health Act
A: allows a social worker to take a person to 'a place of safety'
B: allows a policeman to take any person suspected of suffering from mental illness to a place of safety
C: lasts for 72 hours
D: should be applied so that a mentally disturbed individual can be assessed in hospital
E: should be applied so that a mentally disturbed individual can be assessed by a social worker.

153. In Juvenile delinquency
A: 50% of are likely to re-offend
B: MZ:DZ twin concordance rates are equal
C: inner city adolescents are less vulnerable than rural adolescents
D: the problem is more likely with large family size
E: 20% are marginally mentally retarded

151.

A: **F** There appear to be 2 types: those who are less inhibited who expose themselves with great excitement (20%), and those who are anxious and guilty about their act (80%).

B: **F** 75% are under 40, the peak age being 15-25. If later an associated psychiatric illness (including organic) should be sought.

C: **T** May be underachievers with poor social manner so may give the impression of low intelligence, not confirmed after careful assessment.

D: **T** About 40%.

E: **F** Usually strangers, frequently pubertal girls where the response of disgust is the desired effect. Rape victims are known to the rapist in about 30% of cases.

152.

A: **F**

B: **F** Section 136 allows a policeman to take a person from *a public place* to a place of safety (eg, hospital, police station).

C: **T**

D: **F**

E: **T** The purpose of the section is to allow the individual to be assessed by a psychiatrist *and* an approved social worker who then decide an appropriate course of action (eg, hospital admission, formal or informal).

153.

A: **T**

B: **T**

C: **F** More likely to come from an inner city poor neighbourhood

D: **T** Significantly associated with large family size

E: **F** The majority are of average intelligence but there is a lower mean I.Q. in recidivists.

154. Arson is likely to be repeated if
   A: the offender has a psychiatric history
   B: the offender is psychotic
   C: the offender is mentally subnormal
   D: the offender has a family history of arson
   E: fetishistic excitement occurs

155. Shoplifting
   A: is predominantly carried out by middle aged women
   B: is associated with depression in 30% of cases
   C: is more likely in females who have previous convictions
   D: in males is associated with a higher rate of mental hospital admission than the normal population
   E: is associated with phobic anxiety states

156. Psychopathy
   A: is associated with the chromosomal XYY abnormality
   B: is associated with EEG frontal slow wave abnormalites
   C: requires treatability as a condition of detention
   D: derives from sociopath a term developed by Schneider
   E: is associated with an increased incidence of suicide

154.

A: F Arson is the wilful raising of fire to damage or destroy property and Peak incidence is 17 in men and 45 in women. More common with subnormality and alcoholism. Recurrence more likely if there are multiple attempts, the individual is psychotic, demented, mentally retarded, alcoholic and those who derive sexual excitement from the act.

B: T

C: T

D: F

E: T

155.

A: F Majority in the age range of 10-18.

B: F In the middle aged female group 20-30% may be depressed.

C: F Majority are convicted once and never re-offend.

D: F This has been documented in the middle aged female group but not in males.

E: T

156.

A: T There is a higher incidence of men with XYY abnormality in prisons but the explanations for this remain controversial.

B: F Mainly posterior temporal slow waves.

C: T A recommendation of the Butler report.

D: F Coined by Partridge in 1930.

E: T

157. In the assessment of violence
- A: the presence of morbid jealousy increases the likelihood of repetition
- B: the ability to fantasize decreases the likelihood of enacting violence
- C: a ward nurse can predict better than a doctor
- D: a lack of remorse is a poor indicator
- E: the severity of the act is an indicator of the risk of repeat

158. An interim hospital order
- A: has a maximum period of nine months
- B: after the maximum period a conviction must be recorded
- C: was recommended under the McNaughton Rules
- D: is necessary where the defendant requires medical care during custodial remand
- E: must be followed by a hospital order

159. Testamentary capacity
- A: refers to the capacity to make a valid contract
- B: requires testators consent to be assessed
- C: is absent if a person is deluded
- D: is absent if the patient is detained under the Mental Health Act
- E: requires testator to know the extent of his property in detail

157.

A: T

B: F If associated with a sadistic fantasy life and the collection of weapons may be highly dangerous.

C: F Both are equally liable to error.

D: T

E: T The best predictor appears to be a history of previous violence and the nature of those acts.

158.

A: F 6 months.

B: F The court can decide not to record a verdict.

C: F The Butler committee. The McNaughton Rules were formulated in 1843 following the murder of the then Parliamentary Private Secretary, McNaughton mistaking him for Prime Minister Robert Peel. The rules state that the insanity defence can be invoked where the murderer is incapable of knowing right from wrong and if he does, is unable to see that his act is wrong.

D: T

E: F It can be but it is not mandatory.

159.

A: F Refers specifically to the ability to make a valid will.

B: T Requires that the testator be of 'sound disposing mind'.

C: F A person may be deluded without the delusion influencing him in making the will.

D: F Provided he can express himself 'legibly, clearly and without ambiguity'.

E: F He must understand the act of making a will, know the extent of his property but not necessarily in detail 'and appreciate the claims to which he might give effect'.

SUBSTANCE ABUSE

160. The alcohol dependence syndrome
A: is characterised by salience of drink-seeking behaviour
B: is more common in the offspring of teetotallers
C: is invariably associated with episodes of delirium tremens
D: may not be present in a person with alcoholic cirrhosis
E: was described by Jellinek

161. The following conditions are complications of alcoholism:
A: central pontine myelinolysis
B: Marchiafava Bignami disease
C: Othello syndrome
D: olivo-ponto-cerebellar degeneration
E: lesions in Wernicke's area

162. The following symptoms may result when a person taking 20mgs per day of diazepam stops the drug suddenly:
A: loss of appetite
B: hyperacusis
C: metallic taste in the mouth
D: convulsions
E: auditory hallucinations

160.

A: T Other features are: increased tolerance, withdrawal phenomena, subjective awareness of the compulsion to drink, rapid reinstatement after abstinence, lack of control of drinking and narrowing of drinking repertoire.

B: T

C: F Withdrawal symptoms and subsequent drinking to relieve them is part of the syndrome but does not have to include delirium tremens, a severe withdrawal state with a mortality of around 10%.

D: T It is possible though uncommon through persistent heavy but controlled drinking. Factors which increase the risk of developing cirrhosis include female sex and HLA type.

E: F Edwards and Gross (1976) *Brit Med J,* i, 1058-61.

161.

A: T Especially when hyponatraemia is present.

B: T Demyelination of the corpus callosum, fits and intellectual impairment.

C: T Morbid jealousy.

D: F Autosomal dominant condition.

E: F Wernicke's area (superior temporal gyrus) subserves receptive speech. Not to be confused with Wernicke's encephalopathy - confusion, ataxia, nystagmus and ophthalmoplegias - which is a complication of alcoholism through thiamine deficiency.

162.

A: T

B: T

C: T

D: T

E: F Perceptual disturbances (illusions, micropsia, macropsia) do occur, especially visual. Constitutional anxiety may reappear when benzodiazepines are stopped, but the symptoms described constitute a distinctive withdrawal syndrome. Clonidine, which has been used successfully in treating opiate withdrawal, may prove valuable. (see Petursson and Lader, (1984) 'Dependence on Tranquillisers' Maudsley Monograph, Oxford University Press.)

163. Delirium tremens
  A: occurs in 15% of patients admitted to hospital with alcohol problems
  B: has a peak incidence in the 24 hours after withdrawal from alcohol
  C: may be associated with cross tolerance to benzodiazepines
  D: is associated with respiratory alkalosis
  E: is associated with hypomagnesaemia

164. The following have shown clear efficacy in the treatment of alcoholism:
  A: disulfiram
  B: group therapy
  C: in-patient detoxification
  D: individual counselling
  E: alcoholics anonymous

165. The following are risk factors for the development of alcoholism:
  A: a family history of alcoholism
  B: a family history of depression
  C: a greater preference for spirits than beer
  D: the presence of a phobic disorder
  E: the consumption of 10gm of alcohol a month

163.
A: **F** Occurs in 5% of patients.
B: **F** Peak incidence is 48-96 hours post cessation.
C: **T**
D: **T** Hyperventilation may give rise to alkalosis with elevated pH.
E: **T** May be due to low dietary intake. Decreased magnesium level may lower seizure threshold.

164.
A: **F** None of these have shown to be clearly efficacious. It is likely that the non-specific support provided is the helpful component.
B: **F**
C: **F**
D: **F** Studies have shown that simple advice is as useful as in-patient treatment.
E: **F**

165.
A: **T** Goodwin has demonstrated a significantly higher incidence of alcoholism in adopted away sons of alcoholics compared to adopted away sons of non-alcoholics. Whether this is genetic or environmental is still disputed.
B: **F** There is an increased incidence of depression in families with a history of alcoholism. Despite this, families with a history of depression are not at increased risk.
C: **F** It is the quantity and not the type of alcohol that matters.
D: **F** Secondary alcoholism may occur but is not a risk factor.
E: **F** Even on a daily level this should be safe.

166. Complications of alcoholism include
A: increased incidence of AIDS
B: portal hypertension
C: widening of the gyri of the cerebral cortex on CT scanning
D: raised blood pressure
E: haemochromatosis

167. In chronic cocaine abuse
A: tolerance does not occur
B: dependence may occur
C: prolactin levels may be raised
D: growth hormone levels may be raised
E: formication may occur

168. The following are useful in the management of opiate withdrawal:
A: clonidine
B: naltrexone
C: sodium valproate
D: atenolol
E: chlorpromazine

166.
A: **F** There is an increased incidence of tuberculosis.
B: **T**
C: **F** There is widening of the sulci with narrowing of the gyri. Cerebellar atrophy also occurs.
D: **T** There is increasing evidence that alcohol is a important aetiological factor in hypertension.
E: **F** But the high iron content of some alcoholic drinks along with the hepato-toxic effect of alcohol may exacerbate the condition.

167.
A: **F** Previously cocaine was thought to be an innocuous drug in which neither tolerance nor dependence occurred. The massive upsurge in the use of cocaine in the USA and the evaluation of the problems this has given rise to, has shown this to be false.
B: **T**
C: **F** Many are more likely to be lower.
D: **T**
E: **T** This is a hallucination of touch and takes the form of a feeling that animals are crawling over the body. In cocaine psychoses this occurs along with delusions of persecution and is known as 'the cocaine bug'.

168.
A: **T** Withdrawal symptoms are regularly controlled with methadone but clonidine and naltrexone have recently undergone vigorous evaluation.
B: **T**
C: **F**
D: **F**
E: **T**

MISCELLANEOUS II

169. The risk of coronary heart disease is increased by
A: job dissatisfaction
B: bereavement
C: hyperglycaemia
D: lithium
E: tricyclic antidepressants

170. Erectile impotence
A: is often caused by beta blocking drugs
B: may be treated by antidepressants in certain cases
C: may be caused by a lesion affecting the parasympathetic fibres of the lumbar spinal cord
D: can be treated by the 'squeeze technique'
E: can be treated by the technique of spectatoring

171. Anorexia nervosa
A: is strongly associated with higher social class
B: has a definite genetic component
C: is associated with cystic change in the ovaries
D: occurs in 20% of ballet students
E: is defined as a morbid desire for thinness

169.

A: T So called 'type A' personality. Includes also, competitiveness, drive for success, sense of urgency. In one study risk was almost double in these individuals.

B: T Increased mortality from this and other causes in bereaved spouses (Murray Parkes *et al,* (1969) *BMJ*, i; 740-3).

C: T

D: F

E: F But they may cause fatal cardiac arrhythmias.

170.

A: F Erection (engorgement of the corpus cavernosa) follows parasympathetic stimulation. Ejaculation is mediated by sympathetic fibres and may be delayed by beta blockers.

B: T If depression is the underlying cause. The anticholinergic effects of tricyclic antidepressants may cause impotence.

C: F Sympathetic fibres originate here. Parasympathetic fibres originate in the 2nd, 3rd and 4th sacral spinal segments.

D: F This describes pressure applied just below the glans of the penis which is a technique used to treat premature ejaculation.

E: F Spectatoring is the process in which the subject feels he is an onlooker of his sexual performance. This may cause impotence and is treated by sensate focussing.

171.

A: F Community surveys suggest the social class effect is present but weak.

B: T Twin studies show a significantly higher concordance rate in MZ as opposed to DZ twins, supporting a genetic component to the aetiology.

C: T

D: F Around 7%.

E: F A morbid fear of fatness. Many anorexics do not regard themselves as thin despite obvious emaciation.

172. **Males with eating disorders**
   A: may have abnormalities of the hypothalamic-pituitary-gonadal endocrine axis
   B: have a better prognosis than females
   C: are more common amongst professional jockeys
   D: are 5 times less common than females
   E: are frequently transsexual

173. **The following statements about culture-bound syndromes are true:**
   A: Amok is a condition affecting Malayan women
   B: Latah is a condition of Malayan men
   C: Koro affects males only
   D: Kuru may be due to a slow virus
   E: Windigo is characterised by self-mutilation

174. **Puerperal psychosis**
   A: Is commoner in primiparous women
   B: Is commoner in unmarried mothers
   C: Is commoner following twin delivery
   D: occurs after 1 in 500 births
   E: occurs after 10% of births if the mother has had a previous post-partum psychotic episode.

172.

A: T Similar changes are found to those of women the difference being that the reduced gonadotrophins result in reduced testosterone and hence libido and potency as opposed to amenorrhoea. These are secondary to starvation.

B: F

C: T Analogous to the increased incidence in ballet students.

D: F 10 to 20 times (Beumont *et al,* (1972) *Psychol Med,* 2; 216-31).

E: F May have disturbed sexual identity and orientation but this is not the rule.

173.

A: F Malayan men. After a period of depression and brooding, affected individuals give way to outbursts of uncontrolled rage which usually ends with their suicide.

B: F Malayan women. There are 2 forms: startle reactions and echo reactions. It is a kind of hysterical dissociation.

C: F An acute anxiety state in which the sufferer fears his penis is undergoing fatal retraction into his abdomen. In women, the equivalent fear concerns the nipples or genitalia.

D: F Kuru is due to a slow virus.

E: F North American Indians who believe they have been turned into flesh eating monsters - other people's flesh. Self-biting occurs in the Lesch-Nyhan syndrome, an abnormality of purine metabolism.

174.

A: T May be stress related but metabolic abnormalities such as eclampsia are also more common in the first pregnancy.

B: T

C: F But commoner after difficult pregnancies in general and stillbirth.

D: T 70% affective or schizoaffective, 5-20% schizophrenic and the rest, atypical.

E: T May be even higher. Up to 40% may have a further psychotic episode.

175. **The following may result in clinically significant adverse drug interactions:**
A: lithium and haloperidol
B: clomipramine and tranylcypromine
C: diazepam and atropine
D: guanethidine and phenelzine
E: L-tryptophan and amitriptyline

176. **The following apply to frequency distribution curves:**
A: two standard deviations on either side of the mean will cover 99.8% of the area under a normal distribution
B: the standard error is larger that the standard deviation
C: the standard error is directly proportional to the size of the population
D: in a skewed distribution the median value is a more appropriate measure than the mean
E: kurtosis is related to the shape of a distribution curve

177. **Features of sleep apnoea include:**
A: increased stage 3 & 4 sleep
B: loud snoring
C: night terrors
D: excessive daytime sleepiness
E: family history of the disorder

175.
A: T Isolated cases of neuroleptic malignant syndrome with this combination have been reported.
B: T Contraindicated. Tricyclic/MAOI combinations (such as amitriptyline plus phenelzine) may be used with careful monitoring.
C: F
D: T
E: F May be a beneficial interaction.

176.
A: F Two standard deviations (SD) about the mean covers 96% of the area. 3.09 SD's cover 99.8%.
B: F The standard error of a mean is a measure of the deviation of a sample mean from the true population mean. It may be calculated by dividing the sample variance by the number in the sample and taking the square root.
C: F See above. The square root of the variance is the same as the standard deviation. This is divided by the square root of the number in the sample therefore it is *indirectly* proporional to it.
D: T The median and modal values are less affected by the skew.
E: T Kurtosis refers to the height and width of a normal distribution curve.

177.
A: F Decreases.
B: T Characteristic feature.
C: F These consist of brief episodes of abrupt awakening, occuring during stage 3 and 4 sleep in children.
D: T Due to interruption of stages 3 & 4 nightime sleep.
E: T

178. Chlorpromazine may cause the following side effects:
A: urticarial skin rashes
B: galactorrhoea
C: lens opacities
D: retinal degeneration
E: increase in the seizure threshold

179. In post-natal depression
A: there is a definite genetic component to the milder form
B: psychiatric admission is more likely in nulliparous women
C: psychiatric admission is more likely following caesarian section
D: women in lower social classes are more commonly affected
E: 40% have symptoms after 1 year.

180. In psychiatric disorders affecting women
A: the maternity 'blues' occurs in one third of mothers
B: the maternity 'blues' one week post-partum
C: are more likely to present during the premenstrual period
D: neurotic depression is twice as likely to be diagnosed
E: breast feeding should not be undertaken while receiving antidepressants

178.

A: **T** Remember also photosensitivity rashes.

B: **T** By causing hyperprolactinaemia.

C: **T**

D: **F** This is caused by thioridazine.

E: **F** Lowers the threshold.

179.

A: **F** There is in 'psychotic depression' but not in milder forms.

B: **F** Nulliparous women have had no children so the question is a catch! Admission is more likely in primiparous women.

C: **T** There is an association between caesarian section and admission in the 90 days after delivery.

D: **F** Little evidence to support this. Marital conflict, ambivalence about the pregnancy, difficulties with the pregnancy, increased age and problems with parents are associated.

E: **T** Symptoms include depression, irritability, anxiety and disinterest in sex.

180.

A: **F** Occurs after 50% of births.

B: **F** On the third or fourth day post-partum.

C: **T** Also, an increased incidence of calls to the Samaritans, and their children are more likely to be admitted to hospital during this period.

D: **T** But anxiety and obsessional disorders have an equal sex distribution. Socio-cultural factors are important in referral.

E: **T** Although antidepressants are secreted in small quantities in breast milk, breast feeding is best avoided. Lithium treatment is a contraindication.

SHORT NOTES

(Short Answer Questions)

1. (a) **Outline the production, circulation and absorption of cerebrospinal fluid (C.S.F.).**
(b) **Describe the differences between communicating and non-communicating hydrocephalus.**

Answers
C.S.F. is manufactured by the choroid plexuses of the lateral ventricles by a combination of passive diffusion and active transport. The circulation is as follows: choroid plexuses/ interventricular foramina/3rd ventricle/4th ventricle/foramina of Magendie and Lushka/over the brain stem through the subarachnoid space to the spinal chord and over the cerebral hemispheres. It is absorbed by the arachnoid granulations (villi) into the venous system via the superior sagittal sinus.

Communicating means that dye injected into the lateral ventricles will appear in the subarachnoid space, *ie* that the ventricular system is communicating with the subarachnoid space. Normal pressure hydrocephalus is an example of this.
Non-communicating hydrocephalus is where there is a block between the ventricular and subarachnoid systems, *eg* aqueductal stenosis or tumour in the posterior fossa blocking the 4th ventricle.

2. **Describe the main clinical features of sympathetic and parasympathetic stimulation.**

Answers

Parasympatheric (cholinergic)	Sympathetic (adrenergic)
Small pupils	Large pupils
Exocrine secretion	Dry mouth
Diarrhoea	Sphincter constriction (constipation)
Bronchoconstriction	Bronchodilation
Bradycardia	Tachycardia
Penile erection	Ejaculation
Peripheral vasoconstriction	Vasoconstriction except coronary arteries

119

3. Outline the pathways in the production of the main neurotransmitters.

Answers

Choline acetylase
↓
Choline + acetyl co-enzyme A → *acetylcholine*

Tyrosine hydoxylase   Dopa decarboxylase   dopamine β-hydroxylase
↓   ↓   ↙
Tyrosine → L-Dopa → dopamine → *noradrenaline*

Tryptophan hydroxylase   decarboxylase
↓   ↓
Tryptophan → 5-hydroxytryptophan → 5-hydroxytryptamine (5HT)
                                        (*serotonin*)

Glutamic acid decarboxylase
↓
Glutamate → *GABA*

4. Describe the mechanism of action, indications, precautions and side effects in the use of Monoamine Oxidase Inhibitors (MAOIs).

Answers
Mode of action - increases availability of 5HT and noradrenaline at the post synaptic receptor by inhibiting their degredation.
Indications - resistant and atypical depression, phobic anxiety.
Precautions - interaction with foodstuffs containing tyramine or phenyl-ethylamine (*eg* cheese, chianti wine, Marmite) which are usually destroyed by the gut and liver enzymes. These then enter the systemic circulation producing severe hypertension. Interactions with other drugs especially sympathomimetics.
Side effects - postural hypotension, tremor, oedema, liver toxicity (phenelzine, isocarboxizid), dry mouth.

5. Write short notes on organic hallucinations.

Answers
Visual hallucinations - *eg* small animals, Lilliputian figures as in delirium tremens.
Gustatatory - characteristic of temporal lobe epilepsy (TLE) with uncinate focus.
Tactile (formication) - seen classically in cocaine psychosis associated with delusions of persecution.
Auditory - more typical of functional disorders but can occur in organic states especially temporal lobe lesions. Chronic alcoholic

hallucinosis and patients with long standing TLE may have auditory hallucinations indistinguishable from schizophrenia. *Olfactory* - characteristic of TLE. N.B. local eye or ear disease and drugs (LSD, Cannabis etc) may also be a cause.

6. Describe how one might categorise psychiatric patients seen in a general hospital.

Answers
(a) Physical consequences of psychiatric disturbance (attempted suicide, eating disorders).
(b) Physical illness presenting with psychological symptoms (toxic confusional state).
(c) Somatic symptoms secondary to psychiatric disturbance (abnormal illness behaviour, somatic delusions).
(d) Psychological consequences of physical disease (depression and anxiety in the terminally ill).
(e) Psychological disturbance resulting in poor doctor-patient relationship.
(f) 'Psychosomatic' illnesses (asthma, eczema etc).

7. Describe briefly five defence mechanisms which may operate in psychotherapy.

Answers
1. Projection - externalisation of unacceptable feelings followed by their attribution to others.
2. Displacement - where fear of expressing emotions directly to an individual, leads to their expression to another person.
3. Sublimation - the diversion of instinctual drives towards more socially acceptable outlets.
4. Reaction formation - the acquisition of a trait diametrically opposite to the unacceptable underlying wish.
5. Rationalisation - the attempt to justify actions or desires logically, while remaining unaware of their hidden significance.
   Also, repression, denial and conversion are examples.

8. Outline Piaget's stages of intellectual development.

Answers
After Jean Piaget (1896-1980). Swiss Psychologist.
1. Sensori-motor (birth-2 years) - Object permanence, *ie* knowing things exist even when they are out of view. Differentiation of self from others. Intentionality, *eg* shakes a rattle to make a noise.
2. Pre-operational (2-7years) - Language development and the ability to represent objects by words and/or images. Egocentric thinking, *ie* difficulty taking the other's point of view. Objects classified by a single characteristic.
3. Concrete operational (7-12 years) - More logical about objects and events. Conservation, *ie* the experiment with the long thin glass and the short fat one, accepting that the quantity remains constant when water is transferred from one to the other. Can classify and order objects according to more than one feature.
4. Formal Operational (12years +) - Abstract thinking and can test hypotheses. Concern for morals, rules and the hypothetical.

9. What factors may influence a chronic schizophrenic's course on discharge from hospital into the community.

Answers
Clinical relapse - too rapid discharge without an adequate period of rehabilitation may precipitate relapse. Any change of environment is stressful for such patients.
Premorbid level of adjustment - the quality and quantity of social relationships before the illness must be taken into account, this includes level of employment. For example, a person who was unable to hold down a job before their illness is highly unlikely to be able to afterwards. Sheltered employment is important here.
Loss of skills - secondary to the illness and hospitalisation. Management of finances may be poor because of impaired attention and concentration as well as lack of practice whilst an in-patient. Also, skills learned in hospital generalise poorly in the outside world.
Stigma of mental illness - may lead to homelessness, unemployment, isolation etc.
High expressed emotion - in family environment. Family should be counselled and prepared for the patient's discharge. 'Halfway houses' and hostels may prove less intrusive.

Drug compliance - improved by depot neuroleptics. Regular follow-up by GP or hospital outpatients is required to monitor symptoms and detect early signs of relapse.

10. Outline the principle methods of study in psychiatric genetics.

Answers
Family Studies. The lifetime incidence of a disorder in the relatives of the *proband* is compared to the general population. However, familial aggregation is not proof of genetic factors because of the shared environment.
Twin Studies. Concordance of monozygotic (identical) (MZ) and dizygotic (DZ) co-twins gives a good indication of genetic influences. The most useful comparison is between concordance *rates* of MZ vs DZ twins. The larger this is, the stronger the inheritance. Nevertheless, the shared environment is still uncontrolled in this method of research.
MZ concordance < 100% is due to either environmental factors (upbringing, toxins, infection), modifying genes or reduced penetrance.
Adoption Studies. Rates of illness/trait studied in:-
(a) adopted away offspring of affected parents vs control adoptees
(b) affected adopted away offspring vs sibs remaining in biological family (includes twins)
(c) adopting family of affected individual vs biological family.

11. What considerations go into selecting patients for group psychotherapy.

Answers
An average number of patients is eight. Both sexes should be equally represented. Ideally the age range should be no more than 25 years. Intelligence and educational level should be roughly equal. Care is needed to avoid having only one patient with an outstanding characteristic *eg* homosexual, black, Jewish etc., since this might become unduly focused upon. The patients problems should be diverse unless a group dealing with specific issues is intended e.g victims of sexual abuse, drug addicts etc. Subjects must be able to express ideas and feelings verbally and be prepared to share confidences with the group.
   In general, those with paranoid or marked psychopathic tendencies, psychotics and those with extreme sensitivity, rivalry or narcissism are unsuitable for groups.

12. (a) What are the indications for Electroconvulsive Therapy (ECT)?
(b) What is the Hamilton cuff method?

Answers
The main indication for ECT is to treat a severe depressive illness. Specifically, it is indicated for:- 1. Depressive stupor 2. Delusional depression 3. Retarded depression, especially if the patient is refusing food and drink 4. High suicide risk 5. Antidepressant resistant depression 6. Depression in the elderly and pueperium - particularly effective. 7. Depressive symptoms in dementia and obsessional states, where antidepressants have proved ineffective.

ECT is useful in schizophrenia (catatonic stupor, in combination with phenothiazines where the latter have failed or when affective and schizophrenic symptoms coincide). Also in selected cases of acute mania.

The Hamilton cuff method is used to determine whether a fit has occurred during ECT. A B.P. cuff is inflated to above systolic pressure in one arm after the anaesthetic but before the muscle relaxant. Thus, the effect is seen in the 'isolated' limb, devoid of relaxant.

13. Describe the psychiatric sequelae of head injury. (This could easily be an essay question and may use up a disproportionate amount of time for the unwary. The following layout is recommended).

Answers
Intellectual impairment - related directly to brain damage. Likely to be present if post traumatic amnesia is > 24 hours. More likely if dominant hemisphere. Profound dementia rare.
Personality change - organic and psychogenic factors important, especially after frontal injury. Worse if bilateral, often seen in conjunction with intellectual impairment.
Psychoses - often head injury acts as non-specific stressor. Some evidence that schizophreniform psychosis may be due to specific brain injury (? left sided).
Neuroses - commonest. Depression, anxiety, phobias and obsessional states seen.
Post traumatic syndrome - difficult and much debated topic. Includes headache and dizziness (cardinal symptoms), also fatigue, memory loss and mood changes. May initially be due to

physiological changes but thereafter psychogenic mechanisms predominate. Compensation neurosis may be difficult to distinguish from this. Spectrum ranging from the above to frank malingering (rare).

14. Outline the steps you would take to investigate a man aged 70 presenting with memory loss.

Answers
Substantiate the *history* by interview with an informant - ask specifically about date and speed of onset, mode of progression (gradual, stepwise), history of head injury, drugs (especially alcohol), stroke, high blood pressure. Probe for signs of depression.

Physical and mental state *examination* - look for signs of past cerebrovascular accident, hypertension, gait, primitive reflexes. Mental state for symptoms of depression, psychotic or organic features. Test for recent and remote memory apraxia, aphasia and agnosia. Detailed psychometric testing may be required.
Investigations include routine blood tests especially for vitamin B12, syphilis serology, thyroid function tests. EEG should be performed to look for slow waves. CT scan should ideally be done but not always available.

15. Write short notes on the main psychiatric complications of AIDS.

Answers
Premorbid factors: Homosexuality (if a source of conflict), drug abuse, prostitution.
Bereavement: Terminal illness may provoke depression and/or grief reaction.
Psychosocial: Loss of friends (perhaps through AIDS or fear of AIDS), alteration in life-style, family tension/guilt over homosexuality, unemployment.
Neurotic reactions: Anxiety, obsessional fears/phobias revolving around contamination with virus (usually affects uninfected, low-risk, gay men).
Organic:
(a) Opportunistic infection, eg cerebral toxoplasmosis, cryptococcal menigitits, progressive multifocal leucoencephalopathy.

(b) Primary Human immuno-deficiency virus (HIV) brain disease. Causes a progressive dementia with psychomotor slowing, cognitive defects - especially lack of spontaneity, motivation and poor concentration. Can present with psychosis.
(c) Space occupying lesions, especially CNS lymphomas, cerebral Kaposi's sarcoma.

16. What is Positron Emission Tomography (PET)? Summarise the main findings in:
(a) schizophrenia
(b) affective disorder
(c) dementia

Answers
PET is a techinque which measures the products (positrons) of the radioactive decay of naturally occurring isotopes. They are emitted in an 'annhilation reaction' and are measured outside the skull in slices (tomography). Isotopes can be used to measure blood flow or metabolism and can bind to receptors to estimate receptor density.

(a) Deceased blood flow to frontal lobes (usually bilateral). Chronic populations only. ^{11}C methylspiperone binds to dopamine receptors and may be used to measure receptor density.
(b) Similar 'hypofrontality' in affective disorder. Decreased whole brain metabolism in bipolar depression (depressed phase) which returns to normal with recovery. No consistent changes in unipolar.
(c) Parieto-temporal deficits seen in Alzheimer's disease and decreased frontal lobe metabolism to a lesser extent. Degree of dementia and hypometabolism correlate. Patchy deficits in multi-infarct dementia.

17. Outline:
(a) the main abnormalities found on CT scans in schizophrenic patients
(b) their possible aetiology
(c) their relationship to clinical features

Answers
(a) Enlarged 3rd and lateral ventricles; widened fissures and sulci, found in most studies. Differences due to scan interpretation

(especially planar measurements of scan pictures) and different patient populations.
(b) Twin studies have shown that ventricular size is partly genetically determined. Enlargement commoner in patients without family history and in affected twin in a discordant pair, possibly indicating environmental insult (eg perinatal injury, later mild head trauma with resultant hydrocephalus and infection).
(c) Patients without ventricular enlargement tend to be younger and have less severe illness which responds to treatment. Ventricular enlargement in patients with negative symptoms, cognitive deficits, poor response to treatment and poor premorbid adjustment.
Note, ventricular enlargement also found in manic depressive psychosis.

18. What are the major psychiatric disorders in immigrants to the United Kingdom?

Answers
Schizophrenia - common in Africans, especially with paranoid delusions, religious ideas and hypochondriasis. First rank symptoms (FRS) in 33%. Asians have FRS in 58%. West indians have FRS in 48% with paranoid delusions, religious beliefs and disturbed behaviour common. Atypical psychosis, particularly common in this group, with confusion, paranoid ideas, short duration of illness, good prognosis and negative family history.
Affective disorder - not as common in Africans but may be misdiagnosed. Prominent somatic complaints in Asians. In West Indian, more pronounced sex ratio (ie women>men). Overall, no increased rate but mania significantly increased - ? reaction to stress of migration. Suicide rate lowest in this group.
Neuroses - rates in Africans probably similar to or less than Britons. In Asians, less common than psychoses - somatisation prominent. Evidence conflicting in West Indians, but may be more common than in Britons.

19. (a) What is cognitive therapy?
(b) What are the main stages of the cognitive treatment of depression?

Answers
Cognitive Therapy, as developed by Aaron Beck, is based on the

theory that the way a person interprets his surroundings dictates his reaction to them, and hence his behaviour and mood.

The cognitive theory of depression suggests that abnormal interpretations of the environment result in depressed, negativistic ideas. Cognitive therapy seeks to modify these ideas. There are four main stages:

1. Elicitation of automatic thoughts - in this, thoughts are observed by the therapist which have been spontaneously processed in a negative way (eg the therapist being late means he does not want to treat the patient).
2. Generating alternative ideas - patient is helped to achieve alternative explanations.
3. Reality testing - patient tries out new ideas in practice, often with the aid of a diary.
4. Modification of depressive ideas - relaxation of the patient's cognitive style enables the therapist to modify the underlying depressive assumptions.

20. Discuss the possible neuro-psychiatric complications of volatile substance abuse.

Answers
Up to 10% of boys under the age of 15 experiment with volatile substances in the form of glues, petrol, cleaning solvents, aerosols, paint and lacquer cleaners. Only a small proportion of these abuse solvents regularly. It occurs predominantly in the under 16 age group, twice as common in males compared to females.

Usually undertaken as a group activity, inhalation results in an initial excitatory phase with lack of co-ordination, slurred speech, impaired judgement and a subjective feeling of euphoria and disinhibition. This is followed by a depressive phase with somnolence. Visual and auditory hallucinations have been reported. Acute intoxication may result in coma, epileptic convulsions and sometimes death either due to accidents or to a direct cardio-toxic effect.

Heavy chronic abuse may result in a cerebellar syndrome and rarely an optic or peripheral neuropathy. C.T. scan studies have shown an enlarged ventricular system and widened sulci in long term severe abusers.

The high prevalence of conduct disorder and anti-social personality most likely precedes the abuse of volatile substances. The chronic abuse of volatile substances undoubtedly aggravates the abusers inability to make appropriate psycho-social adjustment.

FURTHER READING

Brain Sciences in Psychiatry. Shaw, DM., Kellam, AMP, Mottram, RE. Butterworth Scientific. 1982. Designed for the old part 1 exam. Patchy but probably the best of its kind.
Child & Adolescent Psychiatry. Eds Rutter, M. Herzov, L. Blackwell. 1985 THE child psychiatry bible. Not light reading.
Companion to Psychiatric Studies. Eds Kendell, RE., Zealley, AK. Churchill Livingstone. 1983. Multi-author Edinburgh textbook. Covers basic science and clinical topics. Very readable especially Kendell's chapters on schizophrenia and affective disorder.
Diagnostic and Statistical Manual (DSM III). American Psychiatric Association. 1980. (DSM IV out soon). Operational criteria for all psychiatric disorders and a useful overview.
Essentials of Postgraduate Psychiatry. Eds Hill, P., Murray R., Thorley A. Grune & Stratton Inc. 1986. Multi-author textbook from the Maudsley. For its size, the most comprehensive book available. Strong bias towards clinical subjects.
Examination Notes in Psychiatry. Bird, J., Harrison, G. John Wright and Sons Ltd. 1984 (regularly updated). Original exam orientated synopsis. Indispensible, lots of good lists!
Fish's Clinical Psychopathology. Hamilton, M. John Wright and Sons Ltd. 1974. Unrivalled synopsis of phenomenology. Must be read! Lots of good German terms.
Handbook of Clinical Adult Psychology. Eds Lindsay, S., Powell, G. Gower. 1987. Brand new and clinically orientated. Recommended.
Handbook of Psychiatry. Ed Shepherd, M. London Institute of Psychiatry. 5 volume authoritative text covering the whole spectrum of psychiatry mainly from a European tradition. Erudite essays not designed for last minute cramming.
Introduction to Psychology. Atkinson, RC., Atkinson, RL & Hilgard, ER, Harcourt Brace Javanovich Inc. 1983. Glossy American text, generously but at times inappropriately illustrated. Theoretical rather than clinical.
Introduction to Psychotherapy. Brown, D., Pedder, J. Tavistock Publications. 1979 Unpretentious and simple account of dynamic psychotherapies.
Manual of Practical Psychiatry. Bebbington, PE, Hill, P. Blackwell. 1985. New book slanted towards management.

Medical Statistics Made Easy. Pipkin, EB. Churchill Livingstone. 1984. Clearly written idiots guide with plenty of examples.
Organic Psychiatry. Lishman, WA. Blackwell Scientific Publications. Second edition 1987. The definitive text on neuropsychiatry. Elegantly written, particularly useful for definition of terms and chapter on head injury.
Oxford Textbook of Psychiatry. Eds Gelder, M., Gath, D., Mayou, R. Oxford University Press. 1983. Clearly written, sensible reference. Needs to be supplemented.
The Scientific Principles of Psychopathology. Eds McGuffin, P., Shanks, MF., Hodgson, MF. Grune & Stratton. 1984. Main rival to 'Companion'. Good chapters on endocrinology, philosophy and genetics.